THE
Fibromyalgia
Cookbook

THE
Fibromyalgia
Cookbook

MORE THAN 140 EASY AND DELICIOUS
RECIPES TO FIGHT CHRONIC FATIGUE

SHELLEY ANN SMITH

FOREWORD BY **ALISON C. BESTED, MD, FRCPC,**
and **ALAN C. LOGAN, ND**

CUMBERLAND HOUSE™

Published by Cumberland House, an imprint of Sourcebooks, Inc.
P.O. Box 4410, Naperville, Illinois 60567-4410
(630) 961-3900
Fax: (630) 961-2168
www.sourcebooks.com

Library of Congress Cataloging-in-Publication Data

Smith, Shelley Ann.
    The fibromyalgia cookbook : more than 140 easy and delicious recipes to fight chronic fatigue / by Shelley Ann Smith.
        p. cm.
    Rev. and updated ed. of: Nashville, TN : Cumberland House Pub., c2002.
    Includes bibliographical references and index.
    1. Fibromyalgia--Diet therapy--Recipes. I. Title.
    RC927.3.S64 2010
    641.5'636--dc22
                    2009050316

Printed and bound in the United States of America.
VP 10 9 8 7 6 5 4 3 2 1

This book is dedicated to the many people who believe in me. My parents—who have always been there for me—for their prayers; my wonderful children and children-in-law Stephen and Kirsten, Kristin and Damon, Adam and Barrett, for their special love and support; and my sisters, Lea, Robin, and Jen. I would also like to dedicate this book to Dr. Cheri Palmer, not only for taking away my pain but also for her continual love, encouragement, and support.

Contents

Foreword

WHAT IS FIBROMYALGIA?

Fibromyalgia (FM) is a chronic musculoskeletal and neurological disorder characterized by widespread pain and tenderness throughout the body. It has been shown to have a genetic predisposition in families. In accordance with the American College of Rheumatology guidelines, the diagnosis of FM is based on a history of chronic widespread pain (on both sides of the body plus above and below the waist) and the finding of at least eleven out of eighteen tender points by a physician (*Arthr. Rheumatol.*, 1990). The diagnosis also includes the following symptoms: fatigue, insomnia, memory and concentration difficulties, sleep disturbance, heart/blood pressure problems, morning stiffness, and gastrointestinal (GI) complaints with potential weight gain.

Chronic Fatigue Syndrome/Myalgic Encephalomyelitis (CFS/ME), a condition where postexertional fatigue is a predominant symptom, is a related and overlapping condition with fibromyalgia.

The definitions of FM and CFS/ME are available online at the National ME/FM Action Network's website at: http://www.mefmaction.net.

Fibromyalgia is not a rare condition; it is, in fact, one of the most common rheumatic illnesses (*Journal of Musculoskeletal Pain*, 2004). A major concern in the field of women's health, FM is prevalent among 6 percent of women, according to the 2003 Canadian Community Health Survey (CCHS). CFS/ME is also prevalent among 3 percent of women in the 2003 CCHS.

Despite volumes of international research, the cause of FM remains unknown. However, we do know that it is a recognized disease. Numerous studies have shown physiological disturbances among FM patients, including hormonal and neurotransmitter abnormalities. Functional MRIs of FM patients' brains show that they react differently than healthy peoples' brains to the same painful stimuli. FM patients are more sensitive to pain after the illness's onset. In fact, FM patients are more sensitive in general—this can include reactions to previously tolerated material, odors, and even food.

To date, research has not revealed a fully effective treatment protocol for FM patients, but there is evidence that low-dose antidepressant medication and carefully monitored exercise programs are of benefit. Recently, investigators have suggested that a multidisciplinary, holistic treatment approach—one that emphasizes education and support—may be the most appropriate. Based on clinical observations and published literature, we believe that proper dietary choices can be a helpful component in FM treatment efforts.

HOW CAN DIETARY CHANGES HELP?

Almost half of all FM patients attempt dietary changes, according to research. Many report this as a helpful approach. Even more encouraging, over 70 percent of CFS/ME patients who attempt dietary change report it as *the most helpful* complementary or alternative intervention. These dietary changes are, however, commonly attempted without guidance and support. Patients are often unaware of alternative choices and meal plans, which usually results in poor compliance beyond the short term.

A number of research papers have shown that vegetarian and vegan diets, at least over the short term, can be beneficial in reducing FM symptoms. In a study published in the *Scandinavian Journal of Rheumatology* (Kaartinen et al., 2000), FM patients on a vegan diet for three months had a 30 percent reduction in tender point numbers and exhibited almost no need for painkillers. Increased intake of fruit and vegetable antioxidant and anti-inflammatory phytonutrients (natural chemicals that give plants their taste, color, and texture) is thought to play a part in the benefit of such diets. This does not mean that FM patients should become vegetarian or vegan; however, it does suggest that reducing proinflammatory animal fat, particularly red meat, and increasing fruits and vegetables may indeed be beneficial.

There is much discussion on the Internet concerning a possible link to nightshade family vegetables and autoimmune diseases (e.g., lupus, rheumatoid arthritis, ankylosing spondylitis). Nightshade vegetables include potatoes, eggplants, tomatoes, and bell/hot peppers, and it has been speculated that these foods might weaken autoimmunity. In recent years this theory has been extended into the realm of fibromyalgia. It is very important to note that there is absolutely no credible research to back up this theory in autoimmunity, let alone fibromyalgia. That said, as clinicians we have observed select patients whose conditions do appear to be aggravated by the aforementioned nightshade vegetables. As with wheat, dairy, and other food groups, the only way to truly identify a nightshade sensitivity is through elimination and challenge. If you find an exacerbation of symptoms with any members of the nightshade family, then by all means eliminate them. However, to give blanket advice to all fibromyalgia patients calling for the elimination of nightshade vegetables is inappropriate. Experimental studies, for example, show that eggplant has anti-inflammatory properties, and tomatoes, eggplants, and bell peppers are all rich in antioxidants— desperately needed antioxidants. If you do have a sensitivity to night-shades then substitute purple cauliflower, cabbage, carrots, and dark green vegetables like spinach, bok choy, and kale, and use sweet pota-toes while avoiding regular spuds.

Another area of recent research involves eliminating food addi-tives such as monosodium glutamate (MSG) and aspartame. In a series of case studies published in the *Annals of Pharmacotherapy* (Smith et al., 2001), eliminating MSG and aspartame led to dramatic improvement in FM symptoms. The investigators reported worsening of symptoms when the patients were challenged with MSG and aspartame. It is possible that MSG, aspartame, and other chemical food additives access the brain through a disturbed blood-brain barrier. The blood-brain barrier is a highly specialized network of blood vessels that normally excludes toxins from the brain. There is emerging evidence that the blood-brain barrier may not be functioning optimally in FM and CFS. Therefore, once inside the nervous system, these synthetic chemicals can act as neurotoxins and disrupt normal transmission between nerve cells. Removing dietary chemical additives has also shown symptom reduction in CFS. Investigators from the University of Newcastle, Australia, reported marked improvements in a number of symptoms, particularly those in the GI tract, when certain food chemicals including MSG were removed. These findings are very important considering that over 70 percent of FM and CFS patients meet the criteria for irritable bowel syndrome during the course of illness.

According to research published in the *Journal of the American College of Nutrition* (October 2001), food intolerances may play a role in the aggravation of FM symptoms. Food intolerances are negative bodily reactions caused by certain foods and are separate and distinct from the classic food allergies. In contrast to a food allergy, where an immediate response is generally observed, the negative reaction to a food may be delayed and take a few days. While classic food allergies to foods such as peanuts and shellfish are relatively rare in the adult population, food intolerances (also called food sensitivities) may be more frequent. Doctors often dismiss the symptoms aggravated by food intolerances, thinking them to be just "in the patient's head." In 2000, a very important paper published in the prestigious journal *The Lancet* challenged this notion. It appears that when patients who are intolerant to foods are challenged with those foods they produce higher levels of inflammatory cytokines—immune chemicals that circulate in the blood. These cytokines can be responsible for the headaches, joint pain, and fatigue observed in FM and CFS/ME. When inflammatory cytokines are purposefully elevated in healthy adults under experimental conditions, the symptoms reported are often quite similar to CFS/ME and FM. Indeed, elevation of these cytokines is even documented to promote symptoms of brain fog, anxiety, and depression in otherwise healthy adults.

While there are a number of methods to determine a food intolerance, the elimination and challenge diet remains the gold standard. Suspect foods—dairy, wheat, citrus, and corn, for example—are eliminated from the diet for a minimum of four days and a maximum of seven days. All of the suspect foods are left out of the diet at the same time. Symptoms may worsen on days two and three as the body goes through a withdrawal of the food. On the fifth day, one of the foods can be introduced back into the diet as part of an elimination-reingestion challenge.

A food diary needs to be kept to record a number of details. The suspected reactions, both physical and emotional, should be recorded before eliminating the suspected food items. The process of reintroducing the food is done one food at a time. This process should always be done the same way. In the morning, take your pulse for a full minute. Record this in the food diary. Eat a small quantity of the challenge food on an empty stomach (see "Testing of Common Problematic Foods" on the next page for sample quantities). Take your pulse before eating the food, then again five, ten, and twenty minutes after eating the food. Record your pulses in your food diary. Also in the food diary, record in a second separate column any physical symptoms such as rash, flushing of your face, heart palpitations, fatigue, or abdominal bloating. In a third column, record any emotional reactions, such as sleepiness, depression, feeling overstimulated, or anxiety. If your pulse rises by ten beats or more, or you have physical or emotional reactions, you may be having an adverse food reaction or a sensitivity reaction to the food in question. Stop the food challenge at that point. Score the severity of the reaction from zero to four. If symptoms occur, they will usually be those that you commonly experience, but they may be more severe than usual. Do not test yourself with foods you suspect you might have an anaphylactic reaction to or worsening of your asthmatic symptoms.

To offset the symptoms such as facial flushing or abdominal bloating, it is sometimes helpful to take one tablet of Alka-Seltzer Gold (United States only) or to take 1 teaspoon of Bisalts (2 parts sodium bicarbonate to 1 part potassium bicarbonate—made by a pharmacist) in a glass of water. This may assist in clearing the reaction more quickly. Symptoms may occur within a few minutes or may take up to twenty-four hours after eating a food that is not tolerated. Do not test another food until the symptoms have cleared completely.

If you do not react to the smallest sample of the food in question, then proceed to the larger portion sizes before your next meal. The testing of various forms of the same food is also important and has been clinically developed by food allergy and intolerance expert Dr. Janice Joneja.

The following are some suggestions.

Testing of Common Problematic Foods

Wheat
Test 1: Puffed wheat or cream of wheat
    (Sample portions: ¼ cup–½ cup–1 cup)
Test 2: Yeast-free cracker
    (Sample portions: 2–4–8 crackers)
Test 3: Regular bread (wheat and yeast)
    (Sample portions: ½ slice–1 slice–2 slices)

Corn

Kernel corn

    (Sample portions: ¼ cup–½ cup–1 cup)

Milk and Milk Products

(Each protein component needs to be tested individually)

Test 1: Casein protein–white cheese, e.g., mozzarella

    (Sample portions: 1 ounce–2 ounces–4 ounces)

Test 2: Casein and whey proteins, e.g., Lactaid milk

    (Sample portions: ¼ cup–½ cup–1 cup)

Test 3: Casein, whey, and lactose, e.g., regular milk

    (Sample portions: ¼ cup–½ cup–1 cup)

Test 4: Casein and modified milk, e.g., yogurt

    (Sample portions: ¼ cup–½ cup–1 cup)

Eggs

Test 1: Egg yolk

    (Sample portions: ½ yolk–1 yolk–2 yolks)

Test 2: Egg white

    (Sample portions: white only of ½–1–2 cooked eggs)

This is a sample elimination diet. More elaborate versions do exist. We recommend performing any elimination and challenge diet under the supervision of a nutritionally oriented doctor or a dietician. Reports in the journal *Neuro-Endocrinology Letters* (2008) highlight the value of supervised elimination diets in CFS symptom reduction. At no time should foods with a previous history of causing a severe anaphylactic or asthmatic reaction be tested unless specifically ordered by your doctor in a medical setting equipped to deal with anaphylactic and asthmatic reactions.

As clinicians we have seen the value of "food as medicine" in many of our patients. Research will undoubtedly continue to uncover the multiple benefits of complex phytonutrients found in fruits, vegetables, and other healthy foods. Since the first edition of this book, emerging studies have shown that patients with FM and CFS/ME are in dire need of a diet rich in antioxidants. It has become clear that FM and CFS/ME patients are under increased oxidative stress where free radical generation is enhanced, and can damage components of the cells within the body, including those mediating pain and/or fatigue. Studies also show that blood levels of protective antioxidant nutrients are low in patients having CFS/ME and FM—almost certainly because they are being "used up" in the defense of the patient's health. Exciting experimental studies have shown that dietary antioxidants have the capacity to reduce pain, fatigue, and even improve mental outlook. Furthermore, new studies have underscored the importance of omega-3 fatty acids and omega-6 fatty acids in FM and CFS/ME. Indeed, much like the antioxidants, there seems to be a stepped-up demand for omega-3 and omega-6 fatty acids by the body in cases of FM and CFS/ME. Levels of these anti-inflammatory fats have been documented to be low in both conditions. Increasing the dietary intake of omega-3 and certain omega-6 oils helps turn down the body's own inflammation pathways and helps therefore to reduce overall body pain in FM and CFS. Increasing dietary intake through oily fish (see www.ewg.org for a list of safe, mercury-free fish) plus nuts (e.g., walnuts contain omega-3 fatty acids) and seeds (ground flax seeds contain omega-3 oils) and supplementing with fish (providing anti-inflammatory omega-3 oils) and evening primrose oils (providing anti-inflammatory omega-6 oils) under the guidance of a professional helps to reduce pain and therefore improve function.

Undoubtedly, research will shed additional light on the reasons why certain foods provoke symptoms in some individuals and why certain chemicals, generally considered safe, may worsen symptoms among patients with FM and CFS/ME. We will expand our knowledge of how dietary fats can either help or harm us, and we will uncover more details on the mechanisms surrounding the ability of dietary antioxidants to provide assistance in the promotion of human health. In the meantime, patients with FM and CFS/ME are suffering in the here and now—and they desperately need guidance. A study published in the *Journal of Human Nutrition and Dietetics* (2009) showed that the majority of patients have unhealthy eating habits—70 percent consuming too many inflammation-promoting dietary fats (too much saturated fat and not enough omega-3), not enough fruits and vegetables, and almost all, 95 percent, with major deficiencies in dietary fiber. FM and CFS/ME patients are often swept up in a vicious circle—the pain and fatigue render the patients unable to spend significant time and energy preparing deeply nutritious meals, and they often skip meals and end up consuming convenient, nutritiously poor meals. The sub-par quality of meals does nothing to promote wellness and pave the road to recovery. In the midst of what seems like a desperate situation, enter Ms. Shelley Ann Smith.

In *The Fibromyalgia Cookbook*, Shelley Ann Smith has provided the instrument needed to increase compliance among those attempting dietary changes. An FM patient herself, Ms. Smith provides a unique perspective on the dietary choices that have helped her in recovery efforts. Knowing how the illness can sabotage the ability, and even the desire, to prepare complex, time-consuming meals, she has provided patients with deliciously simple and quick meals—without compromising even a molecule of vital nutrients. On the contrary, *The Fibromyalgia Cookbook* is stacked from cover-to-cover with nutrient-dense, health-protecting, and recovery-promoting nutrients. She has provided options and alternatives, and most importantly she allows the FM patient or caretaker to choose from a wide variety of foods. One of the realistic concerns of clinicians related to dietary modifications is that if choices are too narrow and limiting, potential nutritional deficiencies could occur. It is essential that FM and CFS/ME patients eat a nutritionally balanced diet with adequate protein, fats, and carbohydrates based on individual caloric needs. This recipe book is not based on a restrictive diet, but rather one that is inclusive of many healthy foods. Ms. Smith recognized a need for support and has filled the void well, hopefully making the lives of fellow-sufferers a little easier. *The Fibromyalgia Cookbook* can be used, along with professional medical guidance, as a means to maintain a healthy diet, one that is so desperately needed when living with a chronic illness.

Enjoy,

Alison C. Bested, MD,
 FRCPC
 Hematological Pathologist
 Medical Staff Liaison
 Environmental Health Clinic
 Women's College Hospital
 Author of *Hope and Help for*
  Chronic Fatigue Syndrome
  and Fibromyalgia
 Toronto, Canada

Alan C. Logan, ND
 Doctor of Naturopathic
  Medicine
 Clinical Consultant
 Author of *The Brain Diet*, *The*
  Clear Skin Diet, and *Your*
  Skin, Younger
 Toronto, Canada

REFERENCES

Altindag, O., Celik, H. Total antioxidant capacity and the severity of the pain in patients with fibromyalgia. *Redox. Rep.* 2006; 11:131–35.

Edman, J. S., et al. A pilot study of elimination/challenge diets in patients with fibromyalgia (FM). *J. Am. Coll. Nutr.* 2001; 19(5):574.

Emms, T. M., et al. Food intolerance in chronic fatigue syndrome. Abstract #15 presented at the proceedings of the American Association for Chronic Fatigue Syndrome conference. January 2001. Seattle, Washington.

Goedendorp, M. M., et al. The lifestyle of patients with chronic fatigue syndrome and the effect of fatigue and functional impairments. *J. Hum. Nutr. Diet.* 2009; 22:226–31.

Gupta, A., et al. Curcumin, a polyphenolic antioxidant, attenuates chronic fatigue syndrome in murine water immersion stress model. *Immunobiol.* 2009; 214:33–39.

Hanninen, O., Kaartinen, K., Rauma, A. L., Nenonen, M., Torronen, R., Hakkinen, S., et al. Antioxidants in vegan diet and rheumatic disorders. *Toxicology.* 2000; 155:45–53.

Haugen, M., Kjeldsen-Kragh, J., Nordvag, B. Y., Forre, O. Diet and disease symptoms in rheumatic diseases—results of a question-naire based survey. *Clin. Rheumatol.* 1991; 10:401–07.

Holton, K.F., et al. Potential dietary links to central sensitization in fibromyalgia: past reports and future directions. *Rheum. Dis. Clin. N. Am.* 2009; 35:409–20.

Hostmark, A. T., Lystad, E., Vellar, O. D., Hovi, K., Berg, J. E. Reduced plasma fibrinogen, serum peroxides, lipids, and apolipoproteins after a 3-week vegetarian diet. *Plant Foods. Hum. Nutr.* 1993; 43:55–61.

Jacobsen, M. B., et al. Relation between food provocation and systemic immune activation in patients with food intolerance. *The Lancet.* 2000; 356(9227):400–401.

Jain, A. et al., Fibromyalgia syndrome: Canadian clinical working case definition, diagnostic and treatment protocols, *Journal of Musculoskeletal Pain* 11, no. 4, 2009.

Joneja, J. V. *Dietary Management of Food Allergies and Intolerances. A Comprehensive Guide.* 2nd edition. J. A. Hall Pub. Vancouver, Canada. 1998.

Kaartinen, K., Lammi, K., Hypen, M., Nenonen, M., Hanninen, O., Rauma, A. L. Vegan diet alleviates fibromyalgia symptoms. *Scand. J. Rheumatol.* 2000; 29:308–13.

Littlejohn, G. Fibromyalgia: What is it and how do we treat it? *Aust. Fam. Physician.* 2001; 30:327–33.

Lukaczer, D., Schiltz, B., Liska, D. J. A pilot trial evaluating the effect of an inflammatory-modulating medical food in patients with fibromyalgia. *Clin. Pract. Altern. Med.* 2000; 1(3):148–56.

Maes, M., et al. In chronic fatigue syndrome, the decreased levels of omega–3 polyunsaturated fatty acids are related to lowered zinc and defects in T cell activation. *Neuroendocrinology.* Letters 2005; 26:745–51.

Maes, M., et al. Normalization of the increased translocation of endo-toxin from gram negative enterobacteria (leaky gut) is accompanied by a remission of chronic fatigue syndrome. *Neuroendocrinology.* Letters 2008; 28:739–44.

Milesi, M., et al. Effect of an oral supplementation with a proprietary melon juice (Extramel) on stress and fatigue in healthy people: a pilot, double–blind, placebo–controlled clinical trial. *Nutr. J.* 2009; 8:40.

Millea, P. J., Holloway, R. L. Treating fibromyalgia. *Am. Fam. Physician* 2000; 62:1575–82.

Nisenbaum, R., Reyes, M., Jones, A., Reeves, W. C. Course of illness among patients with chronic fatigue syndrome in Wichita, Kansas. Abstract #49 presented at the proceedings of the American Association for Chronic Fatigue Syndrome conference. January 2001. Seattle, Washington.

Pioro-Boisset, M., Esdaile, J. M., and Fitzcharles, M. Alternative medicine use in fibromyalgia syndrome. *Arthr. Care Res.* 1996; 9:13–17.

Smith, J. D., Terpening, C. M., Schmidt, S., Gums, J. G. Relief of fibromyalgia symptoms following discontinuation of dietary excitotoxins. *Ann. Pharmacother.* 2001; 35:702–06.

Wolfe, F., et al. The American College of Rheumatology 1990 Criteria for the Classification of Fibromyalgia: Report of the Mulicenter Criteria Committee. *Arthr. Rheumatol.* 1990; 33:160–72.

A Multifaceted Healing Approach

Fibromyalgia is a health issue which for many has a lot of gray areas. As a chiropractor I have found that a multifaceted approach is best. There are four main areas that need to be addressed with someone who has fibromyalgia.

1. **Exercise**. Simple exercise, such as walking, is best as it is low impact, and swimming or biking are great forms of exercise for the same reason. Endorphins are hormones that are released during exercise that reduce pain.

2. **Diet and nutrition**. There are many modifications that can be made to our diets that will reduce pain and inflammation. The following supplements would be very helpful for individuals with fibromyalgia: vitamins E, C, and B; manganese; magnesium; raw veggies; Detox Diet (specifically for liver, kidney, and bowel—reduces toxins that produce inflammation in the body; while reducing red meats and increasing fish and plant oils (omega-3, 6, and 9).

3. **Stress reduction**. Comedy and laughter release endorphins (like exercise) and change mood. Walking in nature or near water will also reduce stress. Yoga and meditation are proven to reduce stress, increase circulation, and give a sense of well-being.

4. **Improved spinal and nervous system function**. As a chiropractor, I see a lot of imbalance within the spine and nervous system with fibromyalgia patients. The human body is a self-regulating, self-healing organism. It is designed to heal itself and regulate all functions. The nervous system runs and controls the whole body and all of its functions. The way we breathe, our digestion, the way we move, our immune system—everything is controlled by the nervous system. As long as there is no interference with this system, one should experience the very best of health. However, with interference, the nervous system will cause malfunction and the body will do its own thing. After the malfunction has been present for a period of time, the body will move into disease mode. Then, the body will speak in the language of symptoms. The symptoms of fibromyalgia are numerous, but the most common include chronic pain, depression, fatigue, muscle stiffness, anxiety, stress, tingling and numbness, neck and back pain, loss of sleep, and bowel problems.

So what can cause interference with the nervous system? Chiropractors call this a vertebral subluxation—this is when one or more of the vertebrae becomes subluxated (misaligned), and this interferes with the way the nervous system controls body functions, including behavior and perception. So quite simply, finding and correcting vertebral subluxations in fibromyalgia patients (as well as many other diseases) will in most cases improve or eliminate the syndrome of fibromyalgia. What causes vertebral subluxations? Emotional stressors (one of the main culprits), physical stress or trauma (accidents, falls, repetitive strain), and chemical stressors (certain foods, alcohol, drugs, toxic chemicals) are the main causes.

Find a good chiropractor in your community who incorporates a multifaceted approach as outlined here—this could change your life or that of someone you love.

Cheri Palmer, BPE, DC

Introduction

On December 5, 1995, my life was radically changed in many unimaginable ways when my youngest son and I were involved in a head-on car accident. We both survived the wreck, and the seemingly harmless surface wounds soon disappeared. Even the nightmares abated after a while. However, my body was shaken to the very marrow of my bones, leaving my defenses at an all-time low, and I became ill with the painful condition called fibromyalgia.

"Fibro" inflicts terrible wounds that leave no scars, and so it is very difficult to explain and much more difficult to treat. Many months went by as I visited doctors for their diagnoses, and the confusion surrounding my problem intensified. Before long it was evident that I would need to alter the very way I live. My career, my lifestyle, my motivations, even my daily tasks and routines all came together for readjustment in a very sobering way. Much courage and trust was needed.

My work experience before the accident included a job as a pharmacy technician. I was well aware of the many drugs available, the pain suppressants, and the myriad of pharmaceuticals. However, my curiosity led me to delve into the natural side of things. I explored healthy alternatives, including herbs and natural foods. I became more aware of the benefits of God's own medicine.

All this knowledge really became beneficial after the accident. Those natural foods and herbs actually helped me and gave me new energy, and I continued to explore the possibilities. I discovered that the old saying "You are what you eat" is poignantly relevant to people suffering with fibro. Their very fabric and fiber are so sensitive and under continual test that any food substances put into their bodies can have intense effects. The solution? Pure foods with no additives, the fewest toxins, and the most nutrition.

Eating the right foods with fibro is not that difficult. You need only to remember a few things and follow a few basic rules. No red meat is easy to remember. Did you know that green peppers contain a compound called solanine, which affects enzyme function in the muscles, causing pain? And that ginger is a powerful antioxidant? We don't eat eggplant and we stay away from heavy, starchy foods because they are hard to tolerate. Our diets are low in sodium, low in fat, with no sugar. But don't worry, sugar lovers, because there are naturally sweet foods we can enjoy, like honey and fruit! We use spelt flour instead of white flour. We love rice pasta and soy butter. We eat extra-virgin olive oil and flaxseed oil on our salads. There are countless possibilities to satisfy every want.

Since publishing the first edition of this cookbook seven years ago, I have only become more convinced of the effectiveness of these dietary changes—from my own experience, yes, but also due to the reader feedback I've received from all over the world. One woman in Canada said, "All the things that I had to learn the hard way (no red meat, no refined flour, no refined sugar, and plenty of fresh raw vegetables) were set out in black and white before me." Partners and family members of those with the disease have found the book useful also, with one man from Australia saying, "Thank you for this great addition to the fight against this chronic disease." And another reader in Kentucky wrote, "I bought the book for a family member with fibro who was nearly an invalid. The improvement was immediate and dramatic. She follows the diet guidelines in the book faithfully and now has her life back." And I've also heard positive feedback from doctors, like this one from Wisconsin who said, "Many of my patients swear by this book and many of my new FMS patients simply swear because they wish that they had found this book sooner." I hope you, too, will come to embrace and trust the recipes I have compiled in this book. I know that all my trusty taste testers—my loving family—have enjoyed helping me.

I want to thank my tasting crew and my family and God for giving me the strength and determination to help me help myself feel better through the ways in which I've altered my life. To the friend of my heart, who with the greatest compassion for my fibro needs and tender love has given me much consolation and support, I say a big thank you!

Turn the page for a recipe to get you started:

Chocolate Soy Smoothie

If you are craving something sweet, blend up a healthy smoothie.

- 1½ cups chocolate soy milk
- 2 bananas
- 2 tablespoons natural peanut butter
- 1 tablespoon liquid honey
- ¼ teaspoon vanilla
- Pinch cinnamon

Blend all ingredients until smooth and frothy.

MAKES 1 SERVING

Basic Guidelines

Water helps with muscle movement, skin tone, digestion, brain function, hair growth, and a whole host of other functions that keep us alive. Filtered, distilled water is your best bet, and the more, the better. Drink at least eight 8-ounce glasses of fresh clean water every day. Drinking so much water may be hard for some people. Try adding a slice of lemon or lime into your water for a refreshing taste. A mint leaf or a slice of orange is also very nice. Remember it is imperative for fibromyalgia sufferers to drink lots of water!

Spelt flour is more than just a nutritious product. The whole-grain flour is the answer for those people who want to eat good, tasty whole-grain products. Spelt is organic, unbleached, and is the grain with most of the bran removed, and nothing added. Spelt contains special carbohydrates that stimulate the body's immune system. One of the most beneficial differences between spelt and wheat is the fact that many wheat- and gluten-sensitive individuals have been able to include spelt-based foods in their diets. It's higher in

B-vitamins and fiber than ordinary bread wheats and has higher amounts of both simple and complex carbohydrates, proteins, and several amino acids.

White flour invokes an inflammatory response in the body, and this causes pain.

Red bell peppers are a better anticancer choice than green peppers because they contain added carotenes. Red bell peppers also have powerful antioxidant properties. Green peppers contain a compound called solanine that affects enzyme function in the muscles, and this causes pain.

Ginger, rosemary, pepper, oregano, and thyme are powerful antioxidants.

Brown rice is high in fiber and can possibly help to lower cholesterol. Brown rice is very high in vitamin B_6 and magnesium. It provides thiamin (which is vital to nerve function), niacin, copper, and zinc. Research studies indicate that vitamin E from brown rice tends to strengthen the immune system and reduce the risk of heart disease and cataracts.

Soy protein is an easy, inexpensive, and healthful alternative to meat. Soy products are dairy-free and do not contain saturated fat.

Stevia is a sweetener made from a natural source ingredient: a shrub native to South America called *Stevia rebaudiana*. 1 package = 2 teaspoons.

Unprocessed food: Eat as much as possible!

Caffeine and sugar: Avoid them!

Low-fat dairy products: Use them!

Red meat: Limit or eliminate!

Soups

Yam-Ginger Soup

This soup is thick and nourishing. If you have a few hours in the morning, you could be enjoying a wonderful soup by lunch time, with some to spare for leftovers. The fresh taste of cilantro and the last-minute addition of cream and black pepper make the wow in this soup. It doesn't matter how you chop the vegetables because they all get blended in the end.

- 1 large onion, chopped
- 2 tablespoons extra-virgin olive oil
- Chicken or vegetable stock
- 3 large carrots, peeled and chopped
- 2 or 3 large yams, peeled and chopped in large pieces
- 2 or 3 cloves garlic, chopped
- 1 tablespoon finely chopped fresh ginger
- ¼ cup fresh chopped cilantro
- Salt and pepper to taste
- Cream or milk, optional

Stir-fry the onion in 2 tablespoons extra-virgin olive oil in large saucepan until soft. Add water and chicken or vegetable stock to half fill pan (add about 2 liters of total liquid). Add rest of the ingredients except cilantro and cream.

Bring to a boil, then gently cook, uncovered, until vegetables are soft.

Blend ingredients until smooth with a handheld processor or mixer.

Add the cilantro.

Serve with a sprinkling of pepper and a few tablespoons of milk or cream.

MAKES ABOUT 8 SERVINGS

Tomato Soup

- 1 onion, chopped
- 3 cloves garlic, finely chopped
- 2 tablespoons extra-virgin olive oil
- 2 cups fat-free chicken broth
- 1 (28-ounce) can chopped tomatoes with herbs and spices
- 1 cup large sourdough croutons

Sauté the onions and garlic in olive oil over medium heat until tender. Do not brown.

Add chicken broth and tomatoes and cook covered for 15 minutes on medium heat. Add croutons and serve.

MAKES 4 SERVINGS

Cauliflower Soup

- 6 cups water
- 1 head cauliflower, cut in small pieces
- 1 medium onion, finely chopped
- 3 tablespoons soy butter
- 1 clove garlic
- ¼ teaspoon pepper
- ¼ cup low-sodium chicken stock
- ¼ cup spelt flour
- 1 cup skim milk

Put 6 cups of water, the cauliflower, onion, butter, garlic, pepper, and chicken stock in a large pot. Bring to a boil. Reduce the heat and simmer until the cauliflower is tender.

Purée the soup in a blender, working in batches if necessary. Return the soup to the pot.

Combine the flour and milk in a medium jar. Shake until smooth. Add the flour mixture to the soup and cook over medium heat, stirring constantly, until the soup thickens.

Bring to a boil and serve.

MAKES 6 SERVINGS

Chilled Cucumber Soup

- 2 cups chopped seeded cucumber
- 1 cup low-sodium chicken broth
- ½ cup low-fat yogurt
- ½ cup low-fat cottage cheese
- 1 teaspoon lemon juice
- ¼ teaspoon Tabasco sauce
- Slivered cucumbers for garnish
- Freshly ground black pepper for garnish

Combine all of the ingredients in a blender and process until smooth. Chill.

Serve in cold soup dishes with slivered cucumbers and freshly ground pepper for garnish.

MAKES 4 SERVINGS

Creamed Carrot Soup

- 2 tablespoons extra-virgin olive oil
- 1 onion, finely chopped
- 10 medium carrots, peeled and chopped
- ¼ cup spelt flour
- 3 cups low-sodium chicken stock
- 1 bay leaf
- 3 tablespoons chopped fresh coriander
- 2 cups skim milk
- Freshly ground black pepper

Heat the olive oil in a saucepan over medium heat and sauté the onion until tender. Add the carrots and cook for 15 minutes.

Sprinkle the flour over the carrot mixture and stir until well blended. Pour the stock slowly into the saucepan, stirring until smooth. Add the bay leaf and coriander, and cook for 20 minutes.

Remove and discard the bay leaf.

Purée the soup in a blender, working in batches if necessary. Return the soup to the saucepan. Stir in the milk and pepper. Cook over low heat until the soup reaches the desired temperature.

MAKES 6 TO 8 SERVINGS

Crabby Clam Soup

- 1 (14-ounce) can Italian stewed tomatoes
- ½ cup grated carrots
- 1 cup finely chopped celery
- 1 cup finely chopped onion
- 1 clove garlic, minced
- Freshly ground pepper
- 1 (6-ounce) tin crab meat with juice
- 1 (10-ounce) can clams with juice
- 2 cups skim milk
- 3 cups water
- ½ cup spelt flour mixed with ½ cup water
- 2 tablespoons low-sodium chicken bouillon powder

Combine the tomatoes, carrots, celery, onion, garlic, and pepper in a large saucepan. Cook over medium heat until tender.

Add the crab meat and clams with their juices, the skim milk, and the 3 cups of water. Mix the flour and ½ cup water in a medium bowl with the chicken bouillon until smooth. Add the mixture to the saucepan and cook, stirring often, until boiling and thickened. Season with pepper to taste. Serve.

MAKES 6 SERVINGS

Mushroom Chowder

- ¼ cup soy butter
- 1 medium onion, finely chopped
- 2 pounds fresh mushrooms, chopped
- ½ cup spelt flour
- 4 cups low-sodium chicken stock
- Fat-free sour cream, optional

Melt the butter in a soup pot over medium heat and sauté the onions until soft. Add the mushrooms and cook for 30 minutes.

Blend in the spelt flour. Slowly add the chicken stock, stirring until smooth. Cover and simmer for 30 minutes.

In a blender purée the soup, working in batches if necessary. Return the soup to the pot and reheat if necessary.

If desired add a dollop of fat-free sour cream to each serving.

MAKES 6 SERVINGS

Lentil Soup

- 1 cup split red lentils
- 3 tablespoons soy butter
- 1 medium onion, finely chopped
- 2 stalks celery, finely chopped
- 2 carrots, finely chopped
- Grated rind of 1 lemon
- 4 cups low-sodium vegetable stock
- Freshly ground black pepper

Rinse and sort the lentils, removing any stones.

Melt the butter in a soup pot over medium heat and sauté the onion until transparent. Add the celery and carrots, and cook for 5 minutes.

Stir in the lentils. Add the lemon rind, vegetable stock, and pepper. Bring the soup to a boil. Reduce the heat and simmer for 20 minutes or until the lentils are tender.

In a blender process the soup briefly, leaving some texture. Return the soup to the pot and reheat if necessary.

MAKES 4 SERVINGS

Split Pea Soup

- 8 cups water
- 2 cups dried split peas
- 4 tablespoons low-sodium chicken stock
- 1 medium onion, finely chopped
- 1 medium carrot, diced
- 1 stalk celery, finely chopped
- 1 tablespoon minced fresh dill
- 2 tablespoons low-sodium soy sauce

Place the water and peas in a large soup pot and bring to a boil. Reduce the heat and simmer for 30 minutes.

Cook the onions, carrots, celery, and dill in a large skillet in the chicken stock until tender.

Drain the peas, reserving the liquid. Add the peas to the skillet with the vegetables and cook for 5 minutes over low heat. Transfer the mixture to the soup pot and add the reserved liquid and the soy sauce. Simmer for 30 minutes.

Purée the soup in a blender, working in batches if necessary. Return the soup to the pot and reheat if necessary.

MAKES 6 TO 8 SERVINGS

Zucchini Soup

- 2 green onions, finely chopped
- 4 tablespoons low-sodium chicken stock
- 2 cups shredded zucchini
- 3 cups skim milk
- 4 tablespoons finely chopped fresh parsley
- 1 teaspoon dried thyme
- ½ teaspoon ground coriander

Cook the onions in a large saucepan in the stock for 4 minutes. Add the zucchini and cook for 5 minutes or until tender. Add the milk, parsley, thyme, and coriander, and bring to a boil. Reduce the heat and simmer for 30 minutes.

Purée the soup in a blender, working in batches if necessary. Return to the pan and reheat before serving.

MAKES 4 SERVINGS

Turkey Bean Soup

- 2 cups low-sodium chicken stock
- 1 cup thinly sliced celery
- 1 cup thinly sliced carrots
- ½ cup finely chopped onion
- ½ teaspoon ground thyme
- ¼ teaspoon dried basil leaves
- Freshly ground black pepper
- 2 cloves garlic, minced
- 1 bay leaf
- 1½ cups cubed cooked turkey
- 3 cups tomato juice
- 1 (15-ounce) can cannellini beans, drained and rinsed

Combine the chicken stock, vegetables, thyme, basil, pepper, garlic, and bay leaf in a large saucepan. Bring to a boil. Reduce the heat and simmer for 15 minutes, and remove the bay leaf. Add the remaining ingredients and simmer until heated.

MAKES 4 SERVINGS

Tomato-Chickpea Soup

- 1 cup dried chickpeas
- 3 tablespoons extra-virgin olive oil
- 2 cloves garlic
- 1½ cups chopped tomatoes
- 3 cups water
- 1 teaspoon dried basil
- 1 chicken bouillon cube
- Freshly ground black pepper
- 1 cup small rice pasta

Put the chickpeas in a bowl of water and soak overnight, covered. Drain and discard the water. Place the chickpeas in a large pan and cover with water. Bring to a boil. Reduce the heat, cover, and simmer for 1 hour until the peas are tender.

Heat the oil in a skillet and sauté the garlic cloves. When browned, remove and discard the garlic. Add the tomatoes and their juice, water, and basil, and simmer for 20 minutes.

Add the drained chickpeas, bouillon cube, and pepper. Stir well and simmer for 10 minutes.

Bring to a boil, add the pasta, and simmer for 10 minutes, or until the pasta is cooked.

MAKES 6 SERVINGS

Sweet Potato Soup

- ¼ cup extra-virgin olive oil
- 2 medium onions, diced
- 3 cloves garlic, minced
- 2 teaspoons thyme
- 3 bay leaves
- 10 cups low-sodium vegetable stock
- 1 cup lentils
- 2 stalks celery, finely chopped
- 1 large carrot, finely chopped
- ½ cup finely chopped fresh parsley
- 2 medium sweet potatoes, peeled and diced
- Freshly ground pepper

Heat the olive oil in a large stockpot over medium heat. Add the onions, garlic, thyme, and bay leaves, and sauté for 10 minutes.

Stir in the vegetable stock, lentils, celery, carrot, and parsley. Bring to a boil. Reduce the heat and simmer uncovered for 40 minutes.

Add the sweet potatoes and cook for 20 minutes. Discard the bay leaves. Season with pepper. Remove 3 cups of the soup and purée in a blender, and return to the pot.

MAKES 4 TO 6 SERVINGS

Cream of Chicken Soup

- 4 tablespoons soy butter
- 8 shallots, thinly sliced
- 2 medium carrots, thinly sliced
- 3 stalks celery, thinly sliced
- 3 boneless, skinless, chicken breasts, finely chopped
- ¼ cup spelt flour
- 5 cups low-sodium chicken stock
- Freshly ground black pepper
- ¾ cup light cream

Melt the butter in a large saucepan over medium-low heat and add the shallots, carrots, celery, and chicken. Cook gently for 10 minutes.

Stir in the flour, blending well. Slowly add the chicken stock, stirring constantly, until smooth. Season with pepper. Cook over low heat for 15 minutes.

Blend in the light cream. Serve.

MAKES 6 SERVINGS

Salads

Tabouli Salad

This is a Middle Eastern recipe that is full of good, healthful ingredients.

- ¾ cup boiling water or chicken stock
- ½ cup cracked wheat
- 1 tomato, diced
- 1 cucumber, seeded and diced
- ½ cup finely chopped green onion
- ½ cup minced parsley
- ¼ cup minced fresh mint leaves
- 3 tablespoons extra-virgin olive oil
- 2 tablespoons lemon juice
- 1 teaspoon sea salt, or to taste
- Freshly ground pepper

Pour boiling water over the cracked wheat. Cover and let stand for 20 minutes until wheat is tender and water is absorbed.

Add the vegetables and chopped herbs and toss to mix.

Combine the oil, lemon juice, salt, and pepper; add to wheat mixture and mix well.

Chill for a couple of hours or overnight for best results.

MAKES 5 TO 7 SMALL SERVINGS

Couscous Salad

A tiny pasta, couscous is small pellets of semolina flour (from the heart of durum wheat). Couscous is thought to date back as far as the tenth century. Whole wheat couscous is available as a recommended alternative to white couscous.

- 2 teaspoons soy butter or margarine
- 3 green onions, chopped
- 1 clove garlic, finely chopped
- 1½ cups water
- ½ teaspoon vegetable or chicken stock granules
- 1 cup uncooked couscous
- 1 tomato, diced
- 1 zucchini, diced
- ¼ cup chopped parsley
- ½ teaspoon dried basil
- ¼ teaspoon pepper

Melt the butter in a saucepan, add the green onions and garlic, and cook until tender.

Stir in the water and stock granules; heat to boiling; remove from heat.

Stir in remaining ingredients.

Cover and let stand 5 minutes or until liquid is absorbed.

Fluff lightly with a fork.

MAKES ABOUT 4 SERVINGS

Beet and Apple Salad

- 1 large beet, cooked, peeled, and grated
- 1 large beet, raw, peeled, and grated
- 2 green apples, thinly sliced

DRESSING

- 4 tablespoons extra-virgin olive oil
- 2 tablespoons lemon juice
- 1 tablespoon finely chopped fresh dill
- Freshly ground pepper

Combine the beets and apples in a salad bowl.

Combine the olive oil, lemon juice, dill, and pepper in a jar. Shake well. Pour the dressing over the beets and apples.

MAKES 4 SERVINGS

Crab Rice Salad

- 1 (6-ounce) can crab, drained
- 1½ cups cooked brown basmati rice
- ¼ cup sliced green olives
- ¼ cup finely chopped celery
- 2½ tablespoons low-fat mayonnaise
- ½ teaspoon finely chopped fresh parsley
- Lettuce, such as iceberg

Combine the first six ingredients in a salad bowl. Mix together, adding more mayonnaise if needed.

Serve over lettuce.

MAKES 4 SERVINGS

Mushroom Salad

- ½ cup extra-virgin olive oil
- 3 tablespoons lemon juice
- 1 tablespoon white wine vinegar
- 1 clove garlic, crushed
- ¼ teaspoon chili powder
- 1 pound fresh mushrooms, thinly sliced
- 1 tablespoon finely chopped fresh chives
- 1 tablespoon finely chopped fresh parsley
- ½ red bell pepper, diced

Combine the olive oil, lemon juice, vinegar, garlic, and chili powder in a jar. Shake and pour over the mushrooms. Toss and chill for 3 hours.

Gently stir in the chives, parsley, and red pepper. Serve.

MAKES 6 SERVINGS

Chicken and Shrimp Salad

- 1 cup cubed cooked chicken
- 1 cup small cooked shrimp
- ½ cup chopped celery
- ½ cup chopped red bell pepper
- ½ cup chopped green onion
- ½ cup low-fat mayonnaise
- 1 tablespoon horseradish
- 1 teaspoon dill weed
- Freshly ground pepper
- 5 cups shredded iceberg lettuce

Combine the chicken, shrimp, celery, pepper, and onion in a medium bowl.

Mix the mayonnaise, horseradish, dill weed, and pepper together in a small bowl. Add to the chicken and shrimp mixture and stir well. Chill for 30 minutes.

Place the lettuce on 4 plates and spoon the salad on top.

MAKES 4 TO 6 SERVINGS

Chicken Salad with Cashews

- 6 boneless chicken breasts, poached and shredded
- 3 celery stalks, cut into thin strips
- 1 large red bell pepper, cut into thin strips
- 3 green onions, sliced
- ½ cup cashews
- 3 cups shredded romaine lettuce

Combine the chicken, celery, red pepper, onions, and cashews in a large bowl. Serve with Mustard Dressing (recipe follows).

Mustard Dressing

- ¼ cup freshly squeezed orange juice
- ¼ cup extra-virgin olive oil
- 1½ teaspoons red wine vinegar
- 1½ teaspoons Dijon mustard
- ½ teaspoon honey
- ½ cup chopped fresh parsley
- Freshly ground black pepper

Combine the ingredients in a blender. Blend well.

MAKES 6 LARGE SERVINGS

Chicken and Tangerine Salad

- 3 chicken breasts, boneless and skinless
- 4 tangerines, peeled and sectioned
- 3 tablespoons chopped pecans
- 3 chives, finely chopped
- 1 tablespoon extra-virgin olive oil
- 2 tablespoons fresh orange juice

Preheat the oven to 350°F.

Place the chicken in a baking dish. Bake for 1 hour.

Cool the chicken and shred into bite-size pieces. Place in a medium bowl and add the tangerine sections, pecans, and chives.

Mix the olive oil and orange juice together in a small bowl. Pour over the salad and toss until coated. Serve at room temperature.

MAKES 4 SERVINGS

Raw Carrot and Green Apple Salad

- 2 green apples, cored and grated
- Juice from 1 lemon
- 2 medium carrots, peeled and grated
- 4 tablespoons extra-virgin olive oil
- 4 tablespoons balsamic vinegar

Toss the apples in a salad bowl with the lemon juice. Mix in the carrots.

Shake the oil and vinegar together in a jar. Pour over the salad and blend.

MAKES 4 SERVINGS

Carrot and Raisin Slaw

- 6 medium carrots, peeled and grated
- ¾ cup diced celery
- ½ cup raisins
- ½ cup diced apple of your choice
- ¼ cup diced onion
- ½ cup low-fat mayonnaise
- Freshly ground pepper

Combine the carrots, celery, raisins, apple, and onion in a medium bowl. Mix in the mayonnaise and season with pepper. Chill.

MAKES 6 SERVINGS

Carrot Salad with Honey Mustard Dressing

- 1 large leek
- 2 tablespoons extra-virgin olive oil
- 6 carrots, peeled and finely julienned
- 1 red bell pepper, seeded and cut into thin strips

DRESSING

- 2 tablespoons red wine vinegar
- 2 tablespoons extra-virgin olive oil
- 2 teaspoons Dijon mustard
- 1 teaspoon honey

Leave 1 inch of green top on the leek and trim off the end. Cut into 2-inch slivers. Wash in several changes of water and dry well.

Heat the oil in a large skillet over medium heat. Add the leek and sauté for 3 minutes.

Add the carrot and red pepper. Cover and cook until crisp-tender.

Prepare the dressing by whisking together red wine vinegar, oil, mustard, and honey in a small bowl. Stir the dressing into the vegetables. Chill for 3 hours before serving.

MAKES 4 SERVINGS

Fresh Citrus-Mint Salad

- 3 large oranges
- 2 white or pink grapefruits
- 8 sprigs mint

Peel the oranges and grapefruits. Separate the sections of fruit. Squeeze the membranes to extract all the juice into a small bowl.

Arrange the segments in a bowl. Chop the mint very finely and stir into the fruit juice. Spoon the juice over the fruit segments and chill.

MAKES 4 SERVINGS

Chicken Waldorf Salad

- ¾ cup low-fat mayonnaise
- 2 tablespoons skim milk
- 2 cups diced apple, such as Spy Apples
- 2 cups diced cooked chicken
- ¾ cup diced celery
- ½ cup chopped walnuts
- ½ cup raisins
- 2 cups shredded lettuce, such as iceberg

Mix the mayonnaise and milk together in a medium bowl. Add the apple and mix. Stir in the chicken, celery, walnuts, and raisins. Blend well together. Spoon the salad over the shredded lettuce.

MAKES 4 SERVINGS

Pink Grapefruit and Scallop Salad

- ¾ cup sea scallops
- 2 pink grapefruits, sectioned
- 1 tablespoon minced chives
- 2 tablespoons grapefruit juice
- 1 tablespoon extra-virgin olive oil
- ½ teaspoon Dijon mustard
- Lettuce leaves, such as iceberg

Cut the scallops in half and cook them in boiling water for 2 to 3 minutes.

Combine the grapefruit sections and chives in a salad bowl. Add the scallops.

Whisk together the grapefruit juice, oil, and mustard in a small bowl. Pour over the scallop mixture and toss well to combine. Serve chilled on lettuce leaves.

MAKES 4 SERVINGS

Jen's Rice and Black Bean Salad

- 1 cup uncooked brown basmati rice
- Low-sodium chicken stock
- 1 (14-ounce) can black beans, drained and rinsed
- 1 large tomato, seeded and chopped
- 1 bunch fresh cilantro, finely chopped
- 3 green onions, chopped
- ½ cup extra-virgin olive oil
- Juice and grated peel of 2 limes

Cook the rice in low-sodium chicken stock according to the package directions and let cool.

Rinse the black beans and add to the rice. Add the tomato, cilantro, and green onions.

Combine the olive oil, lime juice, and lime peel in a small bowl, and mix well. Pour over the rice mixture and stir well. Chill before serving.

MAKES 8 SERVINGS

Pasta Tuna Salad

- 1½ cups brown rice shell pasta
- 1 (8-ounce) can red kidney beans, drained and rinsed
- 1 cup chopped fresh mushrooms
- 1 (14-ounce can) flaked white tuna, packed in water
- ¼ cup chopped fresh chives
- 1 tablespoon dried oregano

DRESSING

- ½ cup extra-virgin olive oil
- 3 tablespoons white wine vinegar
- Juice of 1 lemon
- 1 tablespoon Dijon mustard
- Freshly ground pepper

Cook the pasta shells according to the package directions. Drain and rinse.

Mix the dressing ingredients together in a small bowl.

Mix the pasta, beans, mushrooms, tuna, chives, and oregano in a large bowl. Pour the dressing over the salad and toss to coat. Chill for 1 hour before serving.

MAKES 4 SERVINGS

Pineapple Chicken Salad

- 2 cups diced cooked chicken
- 5 slices fresh pineapple, diced
- 1 banana, sliced
- ¾ cup chopped celery
- ½ cup low-fat mayonnaise
- 2 tablespoons lemon juice
- Salad greens

Toss all ingredients except the salad greens in a large bowl. Line salad bowls with greens and spoon the chicken mixture on top.

MAKES 6 SERVINGS

Zucchini Salad

- 2 cups thinly sliced zucchini
- 4 radishes, julienned
- 1 green onion, chopped

DRESSING

- 6 tablespoons low-fat mayonnaise
- 5 teaspoons skim milk
- ½ teaspoon garlic powder

Toss the zucchini, radishes, and onion together in a salad bowl.

Mix the mayonnaise, skim milk, and garlic powder together in a small bowl. Pour over salad and toss.

MAKES 4 SERVINGS

Salmon Seashell Pasta Salad

- 1 (7½-ounce) can red salmon, drained
- 1 cup small rice pasta seashells
- 1 medium red bell pepper, seeded and cut into slices
- ½ cup thinly sliced celery
- ½ cup diced red onion
- ¾ cup low-fat mayonnaise
- 1 tablespoon white wine vinegar
- 2 tablespoons dill weed

Break the salmon into chunks and set aside.

Cook the pasta in a large pot until tender. Drain well.

Combine the salmon, pasta, red pepper, celery, and red onion in a large bowl.

Whisk together the mayonnaise, vinegar, and dill in a small bowl. Pour the dressing over the salad and toss to combine.

MAKES 4 SERVINGS

Curried Bean Salad

- 1 teaspoon ground cumin
- 2 teaspoons curry powder
- 1 (14-ounce) can kidney beans, drained and rinsed
- 1 red onion, diced
- 2 tomatoes, chopped
- 2 stalks celery, chopped
- 2 green onions, sliced
- 2 tablespoons lime juice
- 1 tablespoon extra-virgin olive oil
- ¼ cup freshly chopped cilantro

Heat the cumin and curry powder in a small skillet and set aside.

Place the kidney beans in a large bowl. Add the onion, tomatoes, celery, and green onions.

Mix the lime juice, olive oil, cumin, and curry powder in a small bowl. Pour over the bean mixture. Stir in the cilantro. Cover and chill, stirring occasionally.

MAKES 4 SERVINGS

Vegetable Turkey Salad

- 2 cups fresh broccoli florets
- 3 cups diced cooked turkey
- 1 medium red bell pepper, seeded and coarsely chopped
- 1 cup fat-free sour cream
- 3 tablespoons low-fat mayonnaise
- 1 tablespoon white wine vinegar
- 1 tablespoon dried basil
- 1 clove garlic, minced
- Freshly ground black pepper

Cook the broccoli until bright green and crisp-tender. Shock in cold water and drain well.

Place the turkey, broccoli, and bell pepper in a salad bowl.

Whisk the sour cream, mayonnaise, vinegar, basil, garlic, and pepper together in a small bowl. Pour the dressing over the turkey and vegetables. Toss gently to coat.

MAKES 4 TO 6 SERVINGS

Fresh Fruit Salad

- ¼ honeydew melon, cut into bite-size pieces
- ¼ cantaloupe melon, cut into bite-size pieces
- 2 peaches, sliced
- 1 banana, cubed
- 2 tablespoons honey
- ½ teaspoon fresh lemon juice

Combine the fruit in a medium bowl. Mix the honey and lemon juice in a small bowl and drizzle over the fruit.

MAKES 4 SERVINGS

Spinach Salad

- 4 cups torn fresh spinach
- ½ cup cubed red bell pepper
- ½ cup thinly sliced red onion, separated into rings
- Favorite salad dressing
- ¼ cup sunflower seeds

Combine the spinach, red pepper, and onion rings in a salad bowl.

Pour on dressing and mix. Sprinkle with sunflower seeds.

MAKES 4 SERVINGS

Tomato and Sweet Pepper Salad

- 3 red bell peppers
- 5 tomatoes, peeled and seeded
- 1 cup sliced cucumber
- 1 clove garlic, minced
- Freshly ground black pepper
- 1 tablespoon extra-virgin olive oil
- 1 tablespoon wine vinegar
- 2 tablespoons chopped fresh cilantro

Cook the peppers on a greased grill over medium heat, turning often, for 20 minutes.

Peel the skin from the peppers. Core, seed, and cut them lengthwise into 1-inch strips.

Cut the tomatoes into thin wedges.

Combine the peppers, tomatoes, cucumber, garlic, and pepper in a salad bowl. Drizzle with the olive oil and vinegar, and toss. Add cilantro and toss. Let stand for 1 hour.

MAKES 4 SERVINGS

Tossed Salad with Sunflower Seeds

- 1 head iceberg lettuce
- 4 tomatoes, chopped
- ½ pound fresh mushrooms
- 1 cup fresh bean sprouts
- ½ cup sunflower seeds
- Favorite salad dressing

Toss all salad ingredients together in a salad bowl and serve with salad dressing.

MAKES 6 SERVINGS

Strawberry Banana Salad

- ½ cup sliced fresh strawberries
- ½ cup sliced bananas
- ½ cup low-fat cottage cheese
- 2 tablespoons plain low-fat yogurt
- 2 tablespoons chopped walnuts
- 4 romaine lettuce leaves, torn into bite-size pieces

Combine the fruit, cottage cheese, yogurt, and walnuts in a small bowl.

Arrange the lettuce in a serving bowl and top with the fruit mixture.

MAKES 1 SERVING

Curry Salad

- 2 (6-ounce) cans shrimp
- 2 cups finely chopped celery
- 1 (10-ounce) can water chestnuts, sliced
- 1 cup fresh bean sprouts
- 2 green onions, chopped
- ¼ cup low-fat mayonnaise
- ¼ teaspoon curry powder

Drain and rinse the shrimp. Transfer to a salad bowl. Add the celery, water chestnuts, bean sprouts, and green onions.

Mix the mayonnaise and curry powder together in a small bowl. Spoon over the shrimp mixture. Toss to coat.

MAKES 4 SERVINGS

Veggies

Bubble Bee Potatoes

This recipe can be modified, perhaps by adding some garlic powder.

- 4 baking potatoes
- ½ teaspoon seasoned salt
- ⅛ teaspoon freshly ground black pepper
- 2 tablespoons extra-virgin olive oil
- 2 tablespoons grated Parmesan cheese
- Salt to taste

Preheat oven to 375°F.

Peel and then wash potatoes.

Cut diagonal slices across the top, only three-quarters of the way through.

Place potatoes on a baking sheet.

Brush with extra-virgin olive oil and season with salt and pepper.

Bake for 1 hour until potatoes are cooked through. I like mine golden brown with a bit of a crunch on the top.

Place potatoes on serving tray and sprinkle with Parmesan cheese.

MAKES 4 SERVINGS

Roasted Parsnips

Roasted parsnips make an ideal addition to pretty much any roasted meat, especially turkey. Best of all, they are so simple to make. Try substituting lemon pepper for regular pepper.

- 1 or 2 large parsnips, peeled
- 5 tablespoons extra-virgin olive oil
- Salt and freshly ground black pepper

Preheat oven to 400°F.

Bring a medium saucepan of salted water to a boil.

Add the parsnips and parboil for 6 minutes.

Place the oil in a roasting pan and put the pan in the oven.

Drain the parsnips and lightly pat dry. Put them in the roasting pan, turning to coat all sides with the hot oil.

Season with the salt and pepper.

Roast for 30 to 40 minutes, turning halfway through cooking time, until golden brown.

Remove from oven and let drain on paper towel to remove excess oil.

MAKES 4 SERVINGS

Grilled Veggie Salad

- 2 large zucchini
- 1 sweet red pepper
- 1 sweet yellow pepper
- 10 medium mushrooms
- 3 tablespoons extra-virgin olive oil
- 2 tablespoons balsamic vinegar
- 2 tablespoons chopped fresh thyme
- 1 tablespoon water
- Seasoned salt and freshly ground black pepper

Cut the zucchini into ¼-inch-thick slices.

Cut peppers in half and remove seeds.

Slice the peppers into ½-inch slices.

Cut mushrooms in half.

Put veggies in large bowl and toss them with 2 tablespoons of oil.

Grill veggies over high heat for 5 minutes on each side or until tender.

Transfer to serving bowl.

Mix together the remaining oil, vinegar, thyme, water, seasoned salt, and pepper. Toss on the hot grilled veggies and enjoy!

MAKES 6 SERVINGS

Balsamic Carrots

- 5 small carrots, peeled and sliced diagonally
- 2 tablespoons balsamic vinegar
- 2 teaspoons honey
- 1 teaspoon extra-virgin olive oil
- ½ teaspoon Dijon mustard
- 1 teaspoon dried basil
- Freshly ground black pepper

Bring 1 cup of water to a boil in a large saucepan and add the carrots. Cover, reduce the heat, and simmer for 10 minutes. Drain the carrots and return to the saucepan.

Combine the remaining ingredients in a small bowl, stirring well with a wire whisk.

Add to the carrots, and cook over medium heat for 5 minutes, stirring often.

MAKES 4 SERVINGS

Parmesan Sautéed Zucchini

- 2 tablespoons extra-virgin olive oil
- 2 cloves garlic, minced
- 2 medium zucchini, cut into thick slices
- Freshly ground black pepper
- Parmesan cheese

Heat the oil in a skillet over medium heat. Add the garlic, and sauté for 2 minutes.

Add the zucchini and cook over medium heat until tender. Season with pepper. Sprinkle with Parmesan cheese.

MAKES 4 SERVINGS

Sesame Green Beans

- 1 pound green beans
- 2 tablespoons sesame seeds
- 1 tablespoon rice wine
- 2 teaspoons low-sodium soy sauce
- 1 teaspoon sesame oil
- Freshly ground black pepper

Trim the green beans. Cook the beans in a large pot of boiling water for 5 minutes or until tender. Drain.

Toast the sesame seeds in a small skillet over medium-high heat, stirring often, until golden.

Combine the rice wine, soy sauce, and sesame oil in a small bowl. Toss with the beans. Add pepper to taste. Sprinkle with sesame seeds.

MAKES 4 SERVINGS

Stir-Fried Squash

- 1 tablespoon extra-virgin olive oil
- 1 clove garlic, crushed
- 1 teaspoon curry powder
- 1 teaspoon freshly grated ginger
- 1 onion, sliced
- 1 winter squash, peeled and cut into large chunks
- 2 tablespoons coriander
- 1 teaspoon low-sodium soy sauce
- Freshly ground black pepper

Preheat the oven to 350°F.

Heat the oil in a skillet or wok and stir-fry the garlic, curry powder, ginger, and onion for 2 minutes.

Add the squash and cook for 5 minutes more.

Roast for 30 minutes in a 350°F oven.

Toss with the coriander and soy sauce. Serve immediately.

MAKES 4 SERVINGS

Sesame Zucchini and Broccoli in Ginger Sauce

- 1 tablespoon extra-virgin olive oil
- ½ head broccoli, cut into florets
- 1 medium zucchini, cut into slices
- Freshly ground black pepper

SAUCE

- 1 tablespoon low-sodium soy sauce
- 1 tablespoon grated fresh ginger
- 1 tablespoon sesame seeds
- 2 teaspoons cornstarch, blended with ½ cup low-sodium vegetable stock

Heat the oil in a large skillet or wok and stir-fry the broccoli and zucchini for 2 to 3 minutes.

Combine the soy, ginger, sesame seeds, and cornstarch mixture in a small bowl. Pour over the vegetables and cook for 3 minutes or until the sauce thickens. Season with pepper.

MAKES 4 SERVINGS

Dilled Mushrooms in Sour Cream

- 1 pound fresh mushrooms
- 3 tablespoons soy butter
- 5 green onions, thinly sliced
- 2 tablespoons spelt flour
- 1 tablespoon fresh squeezed lemon juice
- 2 tablespoons chopped fresh dill
- Freshly ground black pepper
- ¾ cup non-fat sour cream
- Paprika

Clean the mushrooms, pat dry, and quarter.

Melt the soy butter in a large skillet and sauté the mushrooms and onions for 1 minute. Blend in the flour. Add the lemon juice, dill, and pepper. Stir in the sour cream. Heat through. Sprinkle with paprika.

MAKES 4 SERVINGS

Curry Glazed Carrots

- 12 medium carrots
- 2 tablespoons soy butter
- 1 clove garlic, minced
- 1 tablespoon chopped fresh ginger
- 1½ teaspoons curry powder
- 1½ cups low-sodium chicken stock
- 2 tablespoons honey

Peel and cut the carrots into thick slices.

Heat the soy butter in a skillet and sauté the garlic and ginger over medium heat for 1 minute. Add the curry powder and cook for 1 minute.

Add the carrots, stock, and honey, and cook, stirring occasionally, until the liquid evaporates.

MAKES 4 TO 6 SERVINGS

Lemon-Parsley Turnips

- 1 medium turnip, peeled and cut into small cubes
- 2 tablespoons soy butter
- 1 green onion, sliced
- 2 tablespoons chopped fresh parsley
- 2 teaspoons lemon juice

Cook the turnip in boiling water for 15 minutes. Drain.

Stir in the butter, green onion, parsley, and lemon juice. Serve.

MAKES 4 SERVINGS

Asparagus and Cashew Stir-Fry

- 1½ pounds fresh asparagus
- 1 tablespoon extra-virgin olive oil
- 2 teaspoons sesame oil
- 1 tablespoon finely chopped fresh ginger
- ½ cup unsalted cashews
- 1 tablespoon low-sodium soy sauce

Cut the asparagus into 1-inch pieces.

Heat both oils in a skillet. Stir in the ginger and cook for 1 minute.

Add the asparagus and cook until tender.

Stir in the cashews and soy sauce, and cook for 1 to 2 minutes until heated.

MAKES 6 SERVINGS

Sautéed Zucchini and Tomatoes

- 3 tablespoons extra-virgin olive oil
- 4 medium zucchini, sliced
- 1 cup chopped tomato
- 1 clove garlic, minced
- ½ teaspoon dried oregano
- ½ teaspoon dried basil
- Freshly ground black pepper

Heat the olive oil in a large skillet. Add the zucchini and cook until crisp-tender.

Add the tomato, garlic, oregano, basil, and pepper. Cook, stirring frequently, until the zucchini is tender.

MAKES 4 SERVINGS

Baked Yams

- 4 medium yams, peeled and sliced
- 1 cup unsweetened apple juice
- 2 teaspoons freshly grated ginger
- 2 tablespoons honey

Preheat the oven to 425°F.

Combine the yams, apple juice, ginger, and honey in a large bowl. Place in an ovenproof dish and bake uncovered for 30 minutes.

Serve immediately.

MAKES 4 SERVINGS

Garlic Broccoli with Balsamic Vinegar

- 4 tablespoons extra-virgin olive oil
- 1 clove garlic, minced
- 1 bunch broccoli, cut into florets
- Freshly ground black pepper
- 1 tablespoon balsamic vinegar

Preheat the oven to 475°F.

Combine the olive oil and garlic in a small bowl.

Spread the broccoli on a baking sheet. Pour the garlic oil over the broccoli and toss to coat. Season with pepper. Roast for 10 minutes, turning once.

Transfer to a serving dish and sprinkle with vinegar.

MAKES 4 SERVINGS

Fresh Asparagus with Lemon

- 1 bunch fresh asparagus, trimmed
- 2 tablespoons extra-virgin olive oil
- 2 teaspoons lemon pepper
- 1 tablespoon lemon juice
- ½ teaspoon grated lemon zest

Preheat the oven to 475°F.

Spread the asparagus spears on a baking sheet. Pour the olive oil over the asparagus and season with the lemon pepper. Roast for 10 minutes, turning once.

Transfer to a serving dish. Toss with lemon juice and lemon zest.

MAKES 4 SERVINGS

Broccoli with Ginger

- 1 bunch broccoli, cut into florets
- 2 tablespoons extra-virgin olive oil
- 3 teaspoons freshly grated ginger
- 1 tablespoon honey
- 2 tablespoons low-sodium soy sauce
- ¼ cup plus 2 tablespoons water
- 1 tablespoon cornstarch

Steam the broccoli for 5 minutes or until tender.

Heat the olive oil in a medium skillet and sauté the ginger for 1 minute. Stir in the broccoli and cook for 1 minute.

Mix the honey, soy sauce, and ¼ cup water in a small bowl. Pour over the broccoli and cook for another 5 minutes.

Stir in the cornstarch mixed with 2 tablespoons water and cook until thickened.

MAKES 6 SERVINGS

Marinated Tomatoes with Cilantro

- 4 medium tomatoes
- ¼ cup chopped fresh cilantro
- 3 tablespoons extra-virgin olive oil
- 1 tablespoon white wine vinegar
- 1 tablespoon red wine vinegar
- 1 tablespoon dried basil
- ½ teaspoon honey
- Freshly ground black pepper

Slice the tomatoes and arrange on a serving dish. Sprinkle with cilantro.

Whisk together remaining ingredients in a small bowl. Pour over the tomatoes and chill for 1 hour.

MAKES 6 SERVINGS

Stir-Fried Leeks and Snow Peas

- 2 large leeks
- 2 tablespoons extra-virgin olive oil
- 1 medium onion, cut into rings
- 2 cloves garlic, minced
- ½ pound snow peas
- ¼ pound bean sprouts
- 1 tablespoon chopped cilantro
- Freshly ground black pepper

Trim the leeks and cut down the length of one side. Wash thoroughly. Cut the leeks into match-size pieces.

Heat the oil in a large skillet or wok and sauté the onions and garlic for 2 minutes until the onions have softened.

Add the sliced leeks and snow peas, and stir-fry for 4 minutes.

Add the remaining ingredients and cook for 2 minutes. Serve.

MAKES 4 SERVINGS

Dilly Cauliflower

- 1½ cups low-sodium chicken stock
- 2 bay leaves
- 1 teaspoon dill seeds
- 1 head cauliflower, cut into bite-size pieces
- 2 teaspoons Dijon mustard
- 1 teaspoon fresh dill

Pour the chicken stock into a large skillet. Add the bay leaves and dill seeds. Cover and simmer.

Add the cauliflower and simmer until tender.

Chill the cauliflower in its stock for 30 minutes.

Drain, reserving the stock, and place the cauliflower in a serving bowl.

Combine ½ cup of stock with the mustard. Drizzle over the cauliflower and sprinkle with fresh dill.

MAKES 6 SERVINGS

Spinach with Lemon Butter

- 1 pound fresh spinach, cleaned and trimmed
- 2 teaspoons lemon juice
- 2 teaspoons soy butter, melted
- Pinch nutmeg
- Freshly ground black pepper

Rinse the spinach. Cook the spinach in a large saucepan over medium heat for 2 minutes until the leaves have wilted. Drain well.

Sprinkle with the lemon juice, butter, nutmeg, and pepper. Serve.

MAKES 4 SERVINGS

Sautéed Celery

- 1 bunch celery, cut into diagonal slices
- 2 tablespoons extra-virgin olive oil
- 1 bay leaf
- 1 teaspoon dried thyme
- Freshly ground black pepper

Heat the olive oil in a large skillet and cook the celery and remaining ingredients for about 5 minutes.

Discard the bay leaf and serve.

MAKES 4 SERVINGS

Zucchini with Tomatoes

- 1 tablespoon extra-virgin olive oil
- ½ cup finely chopped onion
- 1 cup chopped fresh tomatoes
- 3 cups zucchini, cut into strips

Heat the olive oil in a large skillet and sauté the onion until soft.

Add the tomatoes and zucchini. Cover and cook for 10 minutes. Serve.

MAKES 4 SERVINGS

Ginger Orange Squash

- 3 cups butternut squash, peeled and cubed
- 6 tablespoons orange juice
- 2 teaspoons soy butter
- 1 clove garlic, minced
- 1 teaspoon minced ginger
- Freshly ground black pepper

Combine the squash, orange juice, soy butter, garlic, and ginger in a large skillet over low heat. Cook, covered, over low heat until tender.

Season with pepper.

MAKES 4 SERVINGS

Baked Squash

- 3 acorn squash, cut in half, seeds removed
- 2 tablespoons soy butter
- 2 tablespoons honey
- Freshly ground black pepper
- Sprinkle of cinnamon

Preheat the oven to 375°F.

Place a teaspoon of butter and honey into each squash half. Sprinkle with pepper and cinnamon. Place the squash in a baking dish and cover. Bake for 1½ hours, basting every 15 minutes.

MAKES 6 SERVINGS

Sautéed Cabbage with Caraway

- 1 cup water
- ¾ cup sliced onion
- 4 cups grated cabbage
- 2 tablespoons extra-virgin olive oil
- 1 tablespoon vinegar
- 2 tablespoons caraway seeds

Combine the onion and water in a large skillet. Cover and simmer until onion is soft.

Add the cabbage and stir. Simmer for 10 minutes, or until the cabbage is crisp-tender. Drain and return to skillet over medium-high heat.

Add the olive oil, vinegar, and caraway seeds, and stir-fry for about 5 minutes.

MAKES 4 SERVINGS

Chicken

Grilled Chicken with Peppers

- 4 skinless, boneless chicken breasts
- 6 tablespoons extra-virgin olive oil, divided
- ½ teaspoon dried thyme, divided
- Salt
- 1 red pepper
- 1 yellow pepper
- 2 tablespoons balsamic vinegar
- 1 tablespoon honey
- 2 cloves garlic, minced
- 2 plum tomatoes

Heat BBQ to medium.

Toss the chicken in a large bowl with 2 tablespoons olive oil, half of the thyme, and a pinch of salt.

Slice the peppers in half and core. Brush with 1 tablespoon of olive oil and sprinkle with salt.

Place the chicken and peppers on the grill with the lid closed. Grill for 15 minutes and turn all. Cook until the chicken is fully cooked, about 15 minutes on each side.

Whisk the remaining 3 tablespoons of olive oil in a medium bowl with the vinegar, honey, garlic, and remaining thyme.

Chop the tomatoes and peppers and stir in with other ingredients. Serve over chicken.

MAKES 4 SERVINGS

Stuffed Chicken Breasts

- 1 ounce frozen chopped spinach, thawed
- ½ cup low-fat ricotta cheese
- 2 cloves garlic, minced
- 4 bone-in, skin-on chicken breasts
- Salt and freshly ground black pepper

Preheat oven to 425°F.

Drain the thawed spinach and place in large bowl.

Add the cheese, garlic, 1 teaspoon salt, and ¼ teaspoon pepper. Stir to combine. Set aside.

Loosen the skin on each chicken breast. Place one quarter of the filling underneath the skin of each breast. Press the filling evenly to edges. Season with salt and pepper to taste.

Place on a baking sheet and roast until the chicken is cooked, about 30 minutes.

MAKES 4 SERVINGS

Sesame Chicken Stir-Fry

- 2 tablespoons hot water
- 3 tablespoons dry mustard
- ½ cup low-sodium soy sauce
- 2 tablespoons plus 2 teaspoons toasted sesame seeds
- 1 clove garlic, minced
- 2 tablespoons extra-virgin olive oil
- 4 boneless, skinless chicken breasts, cut into cubes
- Freshly ground black pepper
- 1 tablespoon lemon juice

Combine the hot water and dry mustard in a blender and blend well. Add the soy sauce, 2 tablespoons sesame seeds, and garlic, and blend for 1 minute. Set aside.

Heat the olive oil in a large skillet over medium heat. Add the chicken, season with pepper, and cook until the chicken is done.

Stir in the mustard mixture. Sprinkle with the lemon juice and 2 teaspoons of sesame seeds. Cook for 2 more minutes. Serve.

MAKES 4 SERVINGS

Chicken Chili

- 6 boneless, skinless chicken breasts, cut into ½-inch pieces
- 1 cup finely chopped onion
- 1 cup finely chopped red onion
- 2 medium red bell peppers, chopped
- 2 cloves garlic, minced
- 2 (15½-ounce) cans great Northern beans, drained and rinsed
- 1¾ cups low-sodium chicken stock
- 2 (4½-ounce) cans green chilies, drained and chopped
- ¼ teaspoon cumin

Spray a large skillet with non-stick cooking spray and place over medium heat. Add the chicken, onions, bell peppers, and garlic, and cook until the chicken is done, about 20 minutes.

Add the remaining ingredients and bring to a boil. Reduce the heat and simmer for 10 to 15 minutes or until the sauce thickens.

MAKES 6 SERVINGS

Poppy Seed Mustard-Baked Chicken

- 8 chicken thighs or legs
- 4 tablespoons soy butter, melted
- 4 tablespoons Dijon mustard
- 4 tablespoons honey
- 2 tablespoons fresh lemon juice
- 1 teaspoon paprika
- Freshly ground black pepper
- 3 tablespoons poppy seeds

Preheat the oven to 400°F. Spray a baking sheet with non-stick cooking spray. Place the chicken on the prepared baking sheet.

Combine the soy butter, mustard, honey, lemon juice, paprika, and pepper in a large bowl. Brush the mixture over the chicken. Bake at 400°F for 15 minutes.

Turn the chicken over and brush with the remaining mustard mixture. Sprinkle with poppy seeds. Bake for 15 minutes.

MAKES 4 SERVINGS

Lemon Sesame Chicken

- 4 boneless, skinless chicken breasts
- ½ cup low-fat plain yogurt
- Grated rind and juice of 1 lemon
- 2 teaspoons medium curry paste
- 1 tablespoon sesame seeds

Make cuts in the chicken at intervals with a sharp knife.

Combine the yogurt, lemon rind, lemon juice, and curry paste in a small bowl and whisk to form a smooth mixture. Spoon the mixture over the chicken breasts and arrange them on a baking sheet.

Broil for about 15 minutes, turning once, until the chicken is brown and cooked. Sprinkle with sesame seeds a couple of minutes before taking out of the oven.

MAKES 4 SERVINGS

Tomato-Chicken Casserole

- 2 tablespoons extra-virgin olive oil
- 8 chicken thighs
- 1 medium red onion, sliced
- 2 cloves garlic, minced
- 1 large red bell pepper, cored and sliced thinly
- 1 (14-ounce) can chopped tomatoes
- ½ cup low-sodium chicken stock
- ½ cup thinly sliced sun-dried tomatoes
- Juice and rind of 1 small orange
- 1 tablespoon chopped fresh thyme
- Freshly ground black pepper

Heat the olive oil in a large skillet over medium-high heat and fry the chicken, turning once, until golden brown on both sides.

Transfer the chicken to a large pot. Drain the excess fat from the skillet, add the onion, garlic, and bell pepper, and sauté for 4 minutes.

Transfer the mixture to the pot with the chicken. Add the canned tomatoes, chicken stock, sun-dried tomatoes, and orange juice and rind, and stir to combine. Bring to a boil. Reduce the heat, cover, and simmer over low heat for 1 hour, stirring occasionally.

Add the fresh thyme and pepper before serving.

MAKES 4 SERVINGS

Creamy Chicken Stroganoff

- 3 tablespoons extra-virgin olive oil
- 2½ cups sliced fresh mushrooms
- 2 boneless, skinless chicken breasts, cut into strips
- ½ cup finely chopped onion
- 3 tablespoons spelt flour
- Freshly ground black pepper
- 1 teaspoon paprika
- 1 teaspoon parsley flakes
- 1 tablespoon low-sodium beef bouillon powder
- 1½ cups water
- 1 cup fat-free sour cream
- 2 cups brown rice, cooked

Heat the olive oil in a large skillet over medium heat. Add the mushrooms, chicken, and onion, and cook until the chicken is done, turning once.

Blend in the flour, black pepper, paprika, parsley flakes, and bouillon powder. Stir in the water. Bring to a boil and cook, stirring constantly, until the liquid thickens.

Stir in the sour cream and serve over brown rice.

MAKES 4 SERVINGS

Glazed Chicken with Julienne Vegetables

- 1 (8½-ounce) can low-sodium chicken broth
- ¼ cup apple juice
- 2 tablespoons Dijon mustard
- 2 tablespoons cornstarch
- 1 tablespoon honey
- 2 tablespoons extra-virgin olive oil
- 4 skinless, boneless chicken breasts
- 1 large carrot, cut into thin strips
- 1 medium red bell pepper, cut into thin strips

Stir together the broth, apple juice, mustard, cornstarch, and honey in a small bowl and set aside.

Heat half the oil in a large skillet and brown the chicken. Set aside. In the same skillet heat the remaining oil and stir-fry the carrot and pepper until crisp-tender.

Add the chicken and cover. Continue cooking over low heat, stirring occasionally, until the chicken is fully cooked, approximately 20 minutes.

Stir in the reserved broth/apple juice mixture. Cook until the mixture boils and thickens.

MAKES 4 SERVINGS

Stir-Fried Chicken with Broccoli

- 2 tablespoons low-sodium soy sauce
- 2 cloves garlic, minced
- ¼ cup low-sodium chicken broth
- 4 boneless, skinless chicken breasts, cut into strips
- 1 head broccoli, cut into bite-size pieces
- 2 carrots, cut into strips
- 1 large onion, cut into large slices
- 1 teaspoon Oriental sesame oil

Combine the soy sauce, garlic, and 2 tablespoons chicken broth in a medium bowl. Add the chicken to the broth mixture.

Cook the chicken in a large nonstick skillet with the broth mixture for 5 minutes.

Remove the chicken with a slotted spoon, leaving the liquid in the skillet.

Add the broccoli, carrots, onion, and remaining broth. Cover and cook for 4 minutes.

Add the chicken and cook for 2 minutes. Sprinkle with oil and serve.

MAKES 4 SERVINGS

Red Lentil Chicken Curry

- 2 cups vegetable stock
- ½ cup red lentils, picked over and rinsed
- 2 tablespoons curry powder
- 2 teaspoons ground coriander
- 1 teaspoon cumin seeds
- 8 skinless chicken thighs
- 8 ounces fresh spinach, cleaned well
- 1 tablespoon chopped cilantro
- Freshly ground black pepper to taste

Place the vegetable stock, lentils, curry powder, coriander, and cumin seeds in a large saucepan. Bring to a boil. Reduce the heat, cover, and simmer for 10 minutes.

Add the chicken and spinach and simmer for 50 minutes or until the chicken is done.

Stir in the cilantro and pepper. Serve.

MAKES 4 SERVINGS

Garlic Chicken Breasts

- 4 boneless, skinless chicken breasts
- ½ cup spelt flour
- 1 tablespoon extra-virgin olive oil
- 4 cloves garlic, minced
- ½ cup low-sodium chicken broth
- 3 tablespoons balsamic vinegar
- Freshly ground black pepper
- 1 tablespoon water
- 2 teaspoons cornstarch

Dredge the chicken breasts in flour.

Heat the oil in a large skillet over medium heat. Add the chicken breasts and cook for 3 minutes, turning once. Add the garlic and cook until the chicken is golden.

Add the broth, vinegar, and pepper. Cover and cook at medium heat for 10 minutes, or until the chicken is tender.

Remove the chicken from the skillet.

Mix the cornstarch and water in a small bowl. Add the cornstarch mixture to the skillet and bring to a boil. Cook, stirring constantly, until thickened.

Pour the sauce over the chicken.

MAKES 4 SERVINGS

Honey-Glazed Chicken

- ¼ cup spelt flour
- Freshly ground black pepper
- 4 boneless, skinless chicken breasts
- 3 tablespoons honey
- 2 tablespoons Dijon mustard
- 1 tablespoon extra-virgin olive oil

Preheat the oven to 350°F.

Combine the flour and pepper in a shallow dish. Dredge the chicken breasts with the flour mixture.

Combine the honey and mustard in a small bowl.

Heat the olive oil in a medium skillet over medium heat and brown the chicken on both sides.

Place the chicken on a baking sheet and spread the honey mixture over the chicken.

Bake at 350°F for 15 minutes or until tender.

MAKES 4 SERVINGS

Chicken Breasts with
Toasted Sesame Seeds

- 4 boneless, skinless chicken breasts
- 3 tablespoons extra-virgin olive oil
- ½ cup unsweetened apple juice
- 4 tablespoons chopped green onion
- 4 tablespoons toasted sesame seeds

Heat the oil in a large skillet and brown the chicken on both sides for about 5 minutes.

Add the apple juice and green onion. Simmer for about 20 minutes, until the chicken is cooked.

Place the chicken on a serving platter and spoon the remaining juices over the chicken. Sprinkle with sesame seeds.

MAKES 4 SERVINGS

Baked Chicken Breasts in Yogurt Sauce

- 6 boneless, skinless chicken breasts
- ¼ cup low-sodium chicken stock
- 3 tablespoons Parmesan cheese
- 1½ tablespoons prepared mustard
- 1 teaspoon thyme
- 1 cup low-fat plain yogurt
- 2 tablespoons spelt flour

Preheat the oven to 350°F.

Arrange the chicken breasts in a casserole dish. Combine the chicken stock, cheese, mustard, and thyme in a small bowl. Stir well.

Mix the yogurt and flour together in a medium bowl. Add the cheese mixture. Stir. Spoon the sauce over chicken fillets. Bake uncovered at 350°F for 1 hour or until the chicken is cooked.

MAKES 6 SERVINGS

Chicken and Sweet Pepper Sauté

- 2 teaspoons extra-virgin olive oil
- 4 boneless, skinless, chicken breasts
- 1 red bell pepper, seeded and cut into 1-inch pieces
- 1 yellow bell pepper, seeded and cut into 1-inch pieces
- 1 medium zucchini, sliced
- Freshly ground black pepper
- ¼ cup low-sodium chicken broth
- 4 teaspoons balsamic vinegar

Heat 1½ teaspoons of olive oil in a large skillet over medium heat. Add the chicken and cook until tender and browned on both sides. Remove to a platter.

Add the remaining ½ teaspoon olive oil, peppers, zucchini, and black pepper to the skillet and sauté until tender, stirring frequently.

Add the chicken broth and balsamic vinegar, and bring to a boil.

Pour the sauce over the chicken.

MAKES 4 SERVINGS

Fish

Broiled Flounder with Fresh Basil

- ¼ cup extra-virgin olive oil
- 1 tablespoon lemon juice
- 1 teaspoon chopped fresh basil
- Freshly ground black pepper
- 4 flounder fillets

Preheat the broiler.

Mix the oil, lemon juice, basil, and pepper in a small bowl.

Place the fish fillets in a broiling pan and broil, basting generously with the oil mixture, for 8 minutes or until the fish flakes with fork.

MAKES 4 SERVINGS

Broiled Tarragon Flounder

- ¼ cup extra-virgin olive oil
- 1 tablespoon lemon juice
- 1 teaspoon chopped fresh tarragon
- Freshly ground black pepper
- 4 flounder fillets

Preheat the broiler.

Mix the oil, lemon juice, tarragon, and pepper in a small bowl.

Place the fish fillets in a broiling pan and broil, basting generously with the oil mixture, for 8 minutes or until the fish flakes with fork.

MAKES 4 SERVINGS

Cod with Horseradish Mayonnaise

- 6 tablespoons low-fat mayonnaise
- 1 clove garlic, chopped
- 1 tablespoon chopped cilantro
- 2 teaspoons grated horseradish
- 1 teaspoon grated lemon rind
- Freshly ground black pepper
- 4 (½-pound) cod fillets

Preheat the broiler.

Combine the mayonnaise, garlic, cilantro, horseradish, lemon rind, and pepper in a small bowl.

Grease a broiling pan and place the fish on the pan. Spread the mayonnaise mixture on each fillet. Broil 4 inches from heat for 6 minutes or until the fish is cooked through.

MAKES 4 SERVINGS

Curry Shrimp Skewers

- 1 pound large shrimp
- 4 teaspoons extra-virgin olive oil
- 1 teaspoon curry paste
- ¼ cup finely chopped cilantro

Peel and de-vein the shrimp. Rinse and pat dry.

Stir the oil and curry paste together in a large bowl. Add the shrimp and coat evenly. Cover and refrigerate overnight.

Preheat oven to 375°F.

Place 4 shrimp onto each of 6 skewers.

Place on an oven rack over a baking sheet and bake at 375°F, turning once, for about 5 minutes, until pink.

Transfer to a serving tray. Sprinkle with cilantro and serve.

MAKES 6 SERVINGS

Edwina's Baked Salmon

- 4 (¼-pound) salmon fillets
- ¼ cup low-fat mayonnaise
- ½ teaspoon garlic powder
- ¼ teaspoon pepper
- ¼ teaspoon dill weed

Preheat oven to 450°F.

Place the salmon fillets on greased foil, skin side down. Spread with mayonnaise. Sprinkle with the garlic powder, pepper, and dill weed. Fold the foil over the salmon, sealing completely.

Bake at 450°F for 10 to 15 minutes or until the fish flakes when tested with a fork.

MAKES 4 SERVINGS

Easy Sole Casserole

- 2 tablespoons extra-virgin olive oil
- 1 cup cleaned and sliced fresh mushrooms
- 2 green onions, sliced
- 1 teaspoon dill weed
- ½ teaspoon dried parsley flakes
- 4 sole fillets, cut into bite-size pieces
- ¼ cup fat-free sour cream
- 6 tablespoons low-fat mayonnaise
- 2 tablespoons spelt flour
- Freshly ground black pepper
- Sprinkle of paprika

TOPPING

- 2 tablespoons soy butter
- ½ cup dried brown breadcrumbs

Preheat the oven to 375°F.

Heat the olive oil in a medium skillet and sauté the mushrooms and green onions until tender. Transfer the mushroom mixture to a 2-quart casserole dish and add the dill weed and parsley. Arrange the fish over the mushroom mixture.

Combine the sour cream, mayonnaise, flour, pepper, and paprika in a small bowl. Spread the mixture over the fish.

In a small skillet melt the butter and stir in the breadcrumbs. Stir to coat. Sprinkle the breadcrumbs over the casserole. Bake at 375°F for 30 minutes or until the fish is done.

MAKES 4 SERVINGS

Fillet of Sole with Almonds

- ½ cup spelt flour
- 1 teaspoon lemon pepper
- 4 sole fillets
- 2 tablespoons soy butter
- 2 tablespoons extra-virgin olive oil
- ½ cup sliced almonds
- 2 tablespoons fresh lemon juice
- 1 tablespoon chopped fresh parsley

Combine the flour and lemon pepper on a plate. Dip the fish fillets in the seasoned flour to coat.

Melt 1 tablespoon of soy butter with 1 tablespoon of olive oil in a large skillet over medium heat. Add the fish and cook about one minute per side, or until lightly browned. Remove the fish to a serving plate.

Reduce the heat to medium-low and add the remaining butter and oil. Add the almonds and cook for 2 to 3 minutes. Stir in the lemon juice and parsley. Spoon the almond mixture over the fish.

MAKES 4 SERVINGS

Flounder with Horseradish and Parsley Mayonnaise

- 6 tablespoons low-fat mayonnaise
- 1 clove garlic, minced
- 2 tablespoons chopped fresh parsley
- 2 teaspoons horseradish
- 1 teaspoon grated lemon rind
- Freshly ground black pepper
- 4 flounder fillets

Preheat broiler.

Combine all of the ingredients except the fish in a small bowl. Mix together well.

Grease the broiling pan and place the fish on the pan. Spread the mayonnaise mixture on each fillet.

Broil for 4 to 5 minutes or until the fish is fully cooked and the top is browned.

MAKES 4 SERVINGS

Ginger Shrimp

- 2 tablespoons extra-virgin olive oil
- 1½ pounds fresh shrimp, peeled and cleaned
- 1 inch fresh ginger, peeled and finely chopped
- 2 cloves garlic, finely chopped
- 2 green onions, finely chopped
- ½ cup fresh peas, shelled
- 1 leek, white part only, cut into strips and rinsed
- ¾ cup fresh bean sprouts
- 2 tablespoons low-sodium soy sauce
- 1 teaspoon honey

Heat the oil in a large skillet or wok and stir-fry the shrimp for 2 minutes. Set aside.

Reheat the oil and add the ginger and garlic. Add the onions, peas, and leek. Stir-fry for 3 minutes.

Add the bean sprouts and shrimp to the cooked vegetables. Stir in the soy sauce and honey. Cook for 2 minutes and serve immediately.

MAKES 6 SERVINGS

Orange Roughy with Orange-Lime Sauce

- 4 orange roughy fillets
- ½ cup skim milk
- 6 tablespoons spelt flour
- 2 tablespoons plus 1 teaspoon extra-virgin olive oil
- 1 clove garlic, minced
- 3 tablespoons lime juice
- 2 tablespoons orange juice
- 2 tablespoons finely chopped parsley
- 1 green onion, finely chopped
- 1 tablespoon soy butter

Soak the fillets in milk for 15 minutes.

Dredge the fish in flour, shaking off the excess.

Heat 2 tablespoons olive oil in a large skillet and add the fish. Cook until golden brown, turning once. Remove the fish to a serving platter.

Heat the remaining 1 teaspoon of olive oil in a medium skillet over low heat, add the garlic, and sauté 1 minute. Add the lime and orange juices, parsley, and onion. Add the soy butter and blend well until creamy. Pour the sauce over the fish fillets and serve.

MAKES 4 SERVINGS

Scallops with Citrus Sauce

- 1 tablespoon extra-virgin olive oil
- 1 small onion, finely chopped
- 2 cups large scallops
- 2 tablespoons grated orange rind
- Freshly ground black pepper
- 1 teaspoon dried tarragon
- ¼ cup orange juice
- 1 tablespoon lemon juice
- ¾ cup non-fat sour cream
- 1 tablespoon grated lemon rind

Heat the olive oil in a large skillet and sauté the onion until tender. Add the scallops, orange rind, pepper, and tarragon, and sauté for 2 minutes.

Add the orange and lemon juices, and simmer for 1 minute.

Reduce the heat and stir in the sour cream and lemon rind. Simmer, stirring constantly, for 5 minutes or until the sauce thickens.

Serve with rice or pasta.

MAKES 6 SERVINGS

Scallops with Lemon Pepper Butter

- ¼ cup spelt flour
- 1 teaspoon lemon pepper
- 1 cup fresh scallops
- 4 tablespoons soy butter
- 1 tablespoon fresh lemon juice
- 1 tablespoon chopped fresh parsley

Combine the flour and lemon pepper in a small bowl. Dredge the scallops in the flour mixture.

Melt 2 tablespoons soy butter in a large skillet over medium heat. Add the scallops and cook until golden brown. Remove to a plate.

Reduce the heat, return the skillet to the heat, and melt the remaining butter. Whisk in the lemon juice and parsley. Spoon over the scallops and serve.

MAKES 4 SERVINGS

Sole with Garlic Lemon Butter

- 3 tablespoons soy butter
- 2 cloves garlic, minced
- 2 tablespoons minced fresh parsley
- ½ teaspoon grated lemon rind
- 4 sole fillets
- 2 tablespoons fresh lemon juice

Preheat the broiler.

Cream the butter in a small bowl and blend in the garlic, parsley, and lemon rind. Pat the fish dry. Arrange the fish in a well-greased broiling pan. Sprinkle with lemon juice. Spread with the butter mixture. Broil for 7 minutes or until the fish flakes with fork.

MAKES 4 SERVINGS

Tomato Baked Cod Fillets

- 4 (¼-pound) cod fillets
- 4 fresh tomatoes, cut in half
- 1 tablespoon chopped fresh chives
- 1 teaspoon oregano
- ½ teaspoon dill weed
- ½ teaspoon grated lemon rind
- Freshly ground black pepper
- 2 tablespoons soy butter, melted

Preheat the oven to 400°F.

Spray a shallow baking pan lightly with non-stick cooking spray.

Rinse the fish and pat dry. Arrange the fish in a pan and place tomato halves around the fish. Sprinkle the chives, oregano, dill weed, lemon rind, and pepper over the fish. Drizzle with the melted soy butter. Bake, uncovered, for 20 minutes at 400°F.

MAKES 4 SERVINGS

Tuna Steaks with Ginger

- ¾ cup fresh orange juice
- 1 tablespoon lemon juice
- ¼ cup low-sodium soy sauce
- 1 tablespoon orange rind
- 1 teaspoon chopped fresh ginger
- 1 clove garlic, minced
- 2 tuna steaks

Preheat the broiler or grill.

Combine the citrus juices, soy sauce, orange rind, ginger, and garlic in a shallow baking dish.

Marinate the tuna steaks for 20 minutes. Grill the tuna for 5 minutes on each side, basting with the marinade.

MAKES 2 SERVINGS

Dressings

Fig Dressing

- 3 dried figs, chopped
- 3 tablespoons balsamic vinegar
- 3 tablespoons water
- 2 tablespoons chicken stock
- 2 tablespoons extra-virgin olive oil
- 1½ teaspoons honey
- ½ teaspoon minced shallots
- ½ teaspoon chopped fresh thyme

Combine the figs and vinegar in a saucepan, bring slowly to boil, cover, remove from heat, let stand 15 minutes.

Combine the figs and vinegar with all ingredients in blender and process until smooth.

Yogurt Salad Dressing

- 1 cup low-fat plain yogurt
- 2 tablespoons white vinegar
- 2 tablespoons finely chopped chives
- 2 tablespoons finely chopped parsley
- 1½ tablespoons lemon juice
- Freshly ground black pepper

Combine all of the ingredients in a small bowl and blend well. Refrigerate.

Serve over your favorite salad greens.

Honey Mustard Salad Dressing

- ½ cup non-fat yogurt
- ½ cup low-fat mayonnaise
- ¼ cup honey
- 2 tablespoons lemon juice
- 1 teaspoon dry mustard

Combine all of the ingredients in a small bowl and blend well. Refrigerate.

Serve over your favorite salad greens.

Tarragon Dressing

- ½ cup fat-free sour cream
- ¼ cup low-fat mayonnaise
- ¼ cup skim milk
- 1 tablespoon tarragon vinegar
- ¼ teaspoon crumbled fresh leaf tarragon
- Freshly ground black pepper

Combine all of the ingredients in a small bowl and blend well.

Serve over your favorite salad greens.

Creamy Orange Dressing

- ¼ cup fat-free sour cream
- ¼ cup low-fat mayonnaise
- ¼ cup orange juice
- 1 tablespoon lemon juice
- 2 teaspoons grated orange rind

Combine all of the ingredients in a small bowl and blend well. Cover and refrigerate for up to one day.

Serve over your favorite salad greens.

Curry Salad Dressing

- ½ cup low-fat cream
- ½ cup fat-free sour cream
- 2 tablespoons vinegar
- 1 tablespoon lemon juice
- 2 teaspoons curry powder
- 1 teaspoon honey

Combine all of the ingredients in a small bowl and blend well.

Serve over your favorite salad greens.

Sunflower Seed Salad Dressing

- ½ cup unsalted sunflower seeds
- 1 clove garlic
- Freshly ground black pepper
- 1 tablespoon chopped fresh parsley
- 1 tablespoon lemon juice
- 1 cup plain non-fat yogurt

In a blender process the sunflower seeds. Add the garlic, pepper, parsley, lemon juice, and yogurt to the sunflower seeds and blend until smooth.

Serve as a dip or over your favorite salad greens.

Herbed French Dressing

- 1 cup extra-virgin olive oil
- ¼ cup wine vinegar
- ½ teaspoon seasoned pepper
- ½ teaspoon garlic powder
- ¼ teaspoon dried basil leaves
- ¼ teaspoon dried oregano leaves
- ¼ teaspoon paprika

Combine all of the ingredients in a jar, cover, and shake to combine. Refrigerate.

Serve over your favorite salad greens.

Poppy Seed Dressing

- 3 tablespoons extra-virgin olive oil
- 1 tablespoon fresh lime juice
- 1½ tablespoons honey
- 1 tablespoon water
- 1 tablespoon poppy seeds
- 1 teaspoon grated orange peel

Whisk together all of the ingredients in a small bowl.

Serve with favorite fresh fruit or salad greens.

Yogurt Vinaigrette

- ¾ cup plain low-fat yogurt
- 2 tablespoons white wine vinegar
- 2 tablespoons fresh lemon juice
- 1 clove garlic, minced
- 1 teaspoon Dijon mustard
- Freshly ground black pepper
- 2 tablespoons extra-virgin olive oil
- 2 tablespoons chopped fresh tarragon

Combine the yogurt, vinegar, lemon juice, garlic, mustard, and pepper in a small bowl. Stir well. Stir in the olive oil and tarragon.

Serve over your favorite salad greens.

Lemon Honey Dressing

- ½ cup low-fat mayonnaise
- ½ cup non-fat yogurt
- ¼ cup honey
- 1½ teaspoons lemon juice
- ½ teaspoon dry mustard
- ¼ teaspoon celery seed

Combine all of the ingredients in a small bowl and blend well. Refrigerate.

Serve over your favorite salad greens.

Sauces and Dips

Overnight Salsa

- 1 (2-ounce) package vegetable soup mix
- ⅓ cup boiling water
- 3 large tomatoes, seeded and diced
- ¾ cup canned corn kernels
- ¾ cup rinsed cooked black beans
- ½ cup diced red onion
- 2 tablespoons chopped cilantro
- 1 tablespoon lime juice
- 1 tablespoon extra-virgin olive oil
- 2 teaspoons seeded, finely chopped jalapeño chile
- 1 clove garlic, minced

Combine the soup mix and water in a large bowl. Let stand covered for 10 minutes. Stir in the remaining ingredients, cover, and let stand overnight. This is great served with chicken breasts or rice crackers.

MAKES 3¼ CUPS

Red Bell Pepper Dip

- 1 red onion, unpeeled, halved
- 4 large red bell peppers
- 3 large cloves garlic, unpeeled
- ¼ cup walnuts
- 3 tablespoons Parmesan cheese
- 2 tablespoons red wine vinegar

Preheat the oven to 500°F.

Line a cookie sheet with foil. Place the onion and peppers on the pan. Bake for 20 minutes. Halfway through cooking, add the garlic, and turn the peppers over.

Remove the vegetables from the pan and wrap them in foil, sealing well. Let stand for 10 minutes.

Peel the peppers and take out the seeds. Peel the garlic and onion. Place everything in a blender and add the walnuts, Parmesan cheese, and vinegar. Blend until the mixture is smooth. Chill. Serve with raw veggies.

MAKES 1 CUP

Great Northern Bean Dip

- 1 (15-ounce) can great Northern beans, rinsed and drained
- 2 teaspoons minced fresh thyme
- 2 teaspoons balsamic vinegar
- 1 teaspoon extra-virgin olive oil
- ½ teaspoon dry mustard
- ½ teaspoon ground pepper
- 2 tablespoons minced fresh parsley

Combine the beans, thyme, vinegar, olive oil, dry mustard, and pepper in a medium bowl. Mix with a potato masher until smooth. Stir in the parsley.

Transfer the dip to a serving bowl, cover, and chill for 1 hour. Serve with raw veggies.

MAKES 2¼ CUPS

Creamy Cucumber Dill Sauce

- 1 cup fat-free sour cream
- 1 medium cucumber, peeled, seeded, and shredded
- 3 tablespoons low-fat mayonnaise
- 1 teaspoon dill weed
- 1 teaspoon lemon juice
- Freshly ground black pepper

Combine all of the ingredients in a small bowl. Cover and refrigerate for 1 hour.

Bring to room temperature before serving. Spoon over grilled fish.

MAKES 1½ CUPS

Creamy Parsley Sauce

- ¾ cup fat-free sour cream
- ½ cup low-fat mayonnaise
- 1 tablespoon chopped chives
- 2 teaspoons parsley flakes
- 1 teaspoon dill weed
- 1 teaspoon horseradish
- ½ teaspoon lemon juice
- ½ teaspoon Worcestershire sauce

Mix together all of the ingredients in a medium bowl. Heat the sauce before serving over your favorite fish fillets.

MAKES 1½ CUPS

Pesto Sauce

- 2 cups packed fresh basil leaves
- ½ cup extra-virgin olive oil
- 2 tablespoons soy butter
- ¼ cup pine nuts
- 3 large cloves garlic
- Freshly ground black pepper
- ½ cup fresh grated Parmesan cheese

Combine the basil, oil, soy butter, pine nuts, garlic, and pepper in a food processor and process until puréed. Transfer to a medium bowl. Stir in the cheese. Cover and refrigerate for up to 3 days. Serve with poached, grilled, or baked fish fillets.

MAKES 3 CUPS

Fruit Dip

- 1 cup low-fat yogurt
- 1 tablespoon honey
- Pinch nutmeg
- Pinch allspice

Combine all of the ingredients in a small bowl. Refrigerate. Serve with fresh fruit.

MAKES 1 CUP

Zucchini Dip

- 3 cups shredded zucchini
- ¼ cup finely chopped fresh cilantro
- 3 tablespoons red wine vinegar
- 1 tablespoon extra-virgin olive oil
- 2 cloves garlic, minced
- Freshly ground black pepper
- 3 tablespoons finely chopped pecans

Squeeze the excess water from the shredded zucchini.

Place the zucchini, cilantro, vinegar, olive oil, garlic, and pepper in a blender and process until smooth. Spoon the mixture into a serving bowl and sprinkle with pecans. Chill before serving.

MAKES 3½ CUPS

Dill Dip

- ¾ cup non-fat sour cream
- ½ cup low-fat mayonnaise
- 1 tablespoon onion flakes
- 2 teaspoons parsley flakes
- 2 teaspoons dill weed
- ½ teaspoon paprika

Mix all of the ingredients in a medium bowl. Chill before serving with favorite raw veggies.

MAKES 1½ CUPS

Dill Dip 2

- ¾ cup non-fat sour cream
- ½ cup low-fat mayonnaise
- 3 teaspoons dill weed
- 2 teaspoons onion flakes
- ½ teaspoon celery salt

Combine all of the ingredients in a medium bowl. Chill before serving with raw veggies.

MAKES 1¼ CUPS

Fruit

Fruit Smoothie

- ½ small honeydew melon
- ⅓ cup orange juice
- 1 kiwi, peeled
- Honey to taste

Put all ingredients in blender and pulse until smooth.

Sweeten with honey and enjoy!

MAKES 3 CUPS

Grape Mousse

I love the lightness and the delicate grape flavor of this. There is very little sugar, which makes it appealing to most people. Pure grape juice is best. You can use sweetener in place of the sugar if you wish.

- 2 pouches Knox gelatin
- 2 cups grape juice
- 3 tablespoons sugar
- 1 cup whipping cream
- ½ cup plain yogurt

Put the gelatin into a glass bowl.

Put the grape juice and sugar into a saucepan and cook over low to medium heat until sugar is dissolved.

Pour the juice mixture into the bowl with gelatin. Mix until the gelatin is dissolved.

Whip cream until just before it becomes stiff, then add yogurt and mix.

Divide the juice mixture into 2 bowls. Put whipped cream mixture into one of the separated bowls. Mix well, then pour into a flat serving dish and put in fridge to set, about 3 hours.

Place the rest of the juice mixture on top and again place in the fridge overnight or for several hours before serving.

MAKES 6 SERVINGS

Fresh Fruit Topping

- ½ cup plain low-fat yogurt
- ½ cup low-fat cottage cheese
- 3 tablespoons honey
- 1 teaspoon vanilla extract

Process all ingredients in a blender until creamy. Cover and refrigerate.
  Serve over fresh fruit.

MAKES 6 SERVINGS

Fresh Mangoes with Yogurt

- 3 cups peeled and sliced fresh mangoes
- 8 ounces plain low-fat yogurt
- 1 teaspoon ground cinnamon

Spoon the fruit into chilled fruit bowls. Top with yogurt and sprinkle with cinnamon.

MAKES 4 SERVINGS

Fresh Strawberries with Toasted Coconut

- 2 cups fresh strawberries
- ¼ cup low-fat vanilla yogurt
- 2 tablespoons unsweetened coconut

Toast the coconut in a nonstick skillet over medium heat until lightly browned, stirring constantly, for about 1 minute.

Rinse and clean the berries. Place the berries in a small bowl. Stir in the yogurt. Sprinkle with the coconut.

MAKES 2 TO 4 SERVINGS

Banana Yogurt

- 2 cups chopped bananas
- 1 cup low-fat plain yogurt
- 2 tablespoons honey
- 1 tablespoon lemon juice
- 1 teaspoon grated orange rind

Place all of the ingredients in a blender. Blend until smooth. Chill before serving.

MAKES 4 SERVINGS

Peach Yogurt

- 2 cups chopped fresh peaches
- 1 cup low-fat plain yogurt
- 2 tablespoons honey
- 1 tablespoon lemon juice
- 1 teaspoon grated orange rind

Place all of the ingredients in a blender. Blend until smooth. Chill before serving.

MAKES 4 SERVINGS

Grains

Rice Wraps

Asian, healthy, excellent snack or lunch. This recipe takes a bit more work, so make it on a good day! They can be prepared ahead of time and tightly sealed stored in the fridge for a couple of days. Rice paper wrappers can be found in the Asian section of your grocery store. Soak and work only one rice wrapper at a time, and note that they won't be easy to work with if they absorb too much water.

- Rice paper wrappers
- ¼ cup of cilantro leaves
- ½ cup julienned red peppers
- ½ cup julienned yellow peppers
- 1 cup julienned snowpeas
- 1 (3½ ounce) package enoki mushrooms
- 1 cup bean sprouts
- ¼ cup pickled ginger
- Salt and pepper
- 2 tablespoons black sesame seeds

Fill large bowl with warm water; soak one rice paper wrapper for about 10 seconds or until soft; lay on tea towel to absorb excess water, then transfer to flat surface.

About one third up from the bottom of the wrapper, leaving a 1-inch space on each side, make a line of cilantro leaves, followed by some red and yellow peppers, snow peas, mushrooms, bean sprouts, and a little ginger.

Season to taste with salt and pepper.

Sprinkle top third of the wrapper with sesame seeds.

Carefully fold the bottom of the wrapper over the vegetables; turn in the sides and continue rolling up from the bottom.

To serve, slice roll in half on the bias.

Serve with Orange-Chili Dipping Sauce (recipe follows).

Orange-Chili Dipping Sauce

- ½ cup orange juice
- 3 tablespoons Splenda
- 3 tablespoons soy sauce
- 1 tablespoon balsamic vinegar
- 1 tablespoon sesame oil
- 2 teaspoons lime juice
- 1 teaspoon chili flakes
- 1 teaspoon salt

Whisk together all ingredients in bowl; allow sauce to stand for 30 minutes so flavors can infuse.

Serve at room temperature.

MAKES 1 CUP

Rice Pilaf

- 2 teaspoons soy butter
- ¾ cup chopped pecans
- ¼ cup finely chopped onions
- 1 cup uncooked brown basmati rice
- 2 cups low-sodium chicken broth
- 1 teaspoon dried thyme
- 1 tablespoon chopped fresh parsley
- Freshly ground black pepper

Preheat the oven to 325°F.

Melt 1 teaspoon of soy butter in a medium skillet over medium heat. Add the pecans and sauté for 2 minutes. Remove from the skillet and set aside.

In the same skillet melt the remaining soy butter and sauté the onion until transparent. Add the rice to the onion and stir. Add the chicken broth, thyme, parsley, and pepper. Cover and bring to a boil.

Pour into an ovenproof casserole and bake uncovered until the liquid is absorbed, about 15 minutes, or until the rice is cooked.

Before serving, stir in the pecans.

MAKES 6 SERVINGS

Cilantro Basmati Brown Rice

- 2 tablespoons extra-virgin olive oil
- ½ cup finely chopped onion
- 1 tablespoon finely chopped fresh cilantro
- Dash turmeric
- 1 cup uncooked brown basmati rice

Heat the oil in a medium skillet and sauté the onion until tender. Add the cilantro and turmeric. Stir and set aside.

In a separate pot, cook the rice according to the package directions. Stir the onion mixture into the hot rice.

MAKES 4 SERVINGS

Mushroom Pasta Casserole

- 2 tablespoons extra-virgin olive oil
- 1 clove garlic, minced
- 1½ pounds fresh mushrooms, sliced
- ½ teaspoon basil
- ½ teaspoon thyme
- ½ teaspoon paprika
- 1 teaspoon low-sodium soy sauce
- 3½ ounces Parmesan cheese, grated
- 4 cups pasta sauce
- 1 package rice spaghetti pasta

Preheat oven to 350°F.

Heat the oil in a large skillet and sauté the garlic. Add the mushrooms, basil, thyme, paprika, and soy sauce, and sauté for 15 minutes over low heat.

Place the mushroom mixture in a casserole dish and sprinkle with Parmesan cheese. Cover with pasta sauce. Cover and bake at 350°F for 30 minutes.

Meanwhile, cook the pasta according to the package directions and drain.

Serve the mushroom casserole over the pasta.

MAKES 6 SERVINGS

Pasta with Mushroom Sauce

- ½ pound fresh mushrooms
- 2 tablespoons soy butter
- 2 tablespoons spelt flour
- 1 cup skim milk
- ½ cup fat-free sour cream
- 1 teaspoon ground thyme
- Freshly ground black pepper
- 1½ cups brown rice pasta shells

Clean the mushrooms and chop coarsely.

Melt the butter in a small saucepan and add the mushrooms. Sauté for 5 minutes.

Stir in the flour and cook for 1 minute, stirring constantly. Add the milk, sour cream, thyme, and pepper, stirring constantly. Bring to a boil and cook for 3 minutes.

In a medium saucepan cook the pasta in water until tender. Rinse and drain.

Pour the mushroom sauce over the pasta and serve immediately.

MAKES 4 SERVINGS

Pasta with Basil Sauce

- 1 pound rice pasta, any shape
- 4 tablespoons extra-virgin olive oil
- 2 cloves garlic, minced
- 4 medium tomatoes, peeled, seeded, and finely chopped
- Freshly ground black pepper
- 10 fresh basil leaves, finely chopped

Cook the pasta in boiling water, rinse, and set aside.

Heat the olive oil in a medium skillet and cook the garlic and tomatoes with pepper over medium heat for 10 minutes.

Stir the well-drained pasta into the skillet and mix well until heated.

Sprinkle chopped basil leaves over the pasta before serving.

MAKES 4 SERVINGS

Pasta with Pesto Sauce

- 2 cups rice pasta
- 2 cups fresh basil
- 3 tablespoons pine nuts
- 3 cloves garlic, chopped
- Freshly ground black pepper
- ½ cup extra-virgin olive oil
- ¼ cup Parmesan cheese

Cook the pasta in a large pot of boiling water until tender. Drain and return to the pot.

Process the basil, pine nuts, garlic, and pepper in a blender until smooth.

Slowly add the olive oil and Parmesan cheese, blending well.

Pour the pesto sauce over the pasta and coat well.

MAKES 6 SERVINGS

Oatmeal Pancakes

What a way to start your day with these healthful pancakes. I make a whole batch at once, then I store them in the fridge and can pull some out anytime to toast and enjoy.

- 1 cup oatmeal, or oatmeal mix (see recipe in this book)
- 2 cups buttermilk
- 2 eggs
- 3 tablespoons sugar substitute or brown sugar
- 1 tablespoon vegetable oil
- 1 teaspoon vanilla
- 1½ cups spelt flour
- 1 teaspoon baking powder
- 1 teaspoon baking soda
- ½ teaspoon salt
- 1 teaspoon cinnamon

Combine oat mixture, or oats, with buttermilk in large bowl and let sit for 2 minutes.

Add the eggs, sugar substitute or brown sugar, vegetable oil, and vanilla and stir well.

Combine flour, baking powder, baking soda, salt, and cinnamon in a small bowl.

Add dry mixture to wet in the large bowl, stir only enough to mix.

Coat a frying pan or pancake pan with small amount of oil to avoid sticking. You may use a non-stick pan. Spoon small amounts of mixture to make 4-inch pancakes. When bubbles appear and break on top of pancakes, flip them over.

Enjoy with fresh fruit.

MAKES 12 SMALL PANCAKES

Lea's Oat Mixture

I compiled this tasty cereal combination and haven't looked back since. I use it often as a hot cereal and as filler ingredients for oat pancakes, muffins, and breads. This recipe can be halved, some other ingredients added, or some removed. You will need a very large bowl for mixing if you do the full-scale version.

- 12 cups quick oats
- 6 cups large flake oats
- 2 cups cracked wheat
- 3 cups wheat bran
- 3 cups oat bran
- 2 cups wheat germ
- 2 cups crushed flaxseed
- 2 cups walnuts, chopped small

Mix and store in airtight container.

Breads

Raisin Loaf

- 1 cup honey
- 1 cup skim milk
- 1 cup raisins
- ½ cup Becel olive oil margarine
- 1 teaspoon vanilla
- ½ teaspoon ground cinnamon
- ¼ teaspoon salt
- ¼ teaspoon ground nutmeg
- ¼ teaspoon ground cloves
- 3 cups spelt flour
- 1 teaspoon baking powder
- ½ teaspoon baking soda
- ½ cup walnuts, optional

Preheat the oven to 350°F.

Place the honey, milk, raisins, margarine, vanilla, cinnamon, salt, nutmeg, and cloves in a large sauce pan over medium heat and boil for 8 minutes. Transfer to large bowl to cool for 10 minutes

Mix the flour, baking powder, and baking soda in a bowl and mix into wet ingredients. Add the walnuts if desired. Put dough in a greased loaf pan and bake at 350°F for 45 minutes.

Flaxseed Muffins

The tiny flax seed is loaded with nutritional benefits such as soluble fiber and heart-healthy omega-3 fatty acid. These muffins pack a punch of goodness with the carrots, apples, and bran and without any cooking oil of any kind!

- 1½ cups spelt flour
- 1 cup brown sugar
- ¾ cup crushed flaxseed
- ¾ cup oat bran
- 2 teaspoons baking soda
- 2 teaspoons cinnamon
- 1 teaspoon baking powder
- ½ teaspoon salt
- 1½ cups shredded carrots
- 2 peeled and shredded apples of your choice
- 1 cup chopped nuts
- ½ cup raisins, optional
- ¾ cup milk
- 2 beaten eggs
- 1 teaspoon vanilla

Preheat oven to 350°F.

Mix together flour, brown sugar, flaxseed, oat bran, baking soda, cinnamon, baking powder, and salt in a large bowl.

Stir in carrots, apples, nuts, and raisins, if desired.

Combine milk, beaten eggs, and vanilla. Pour liquid into dry ingredients. Stir until moistened only. Do not overmix.

Place muffin cups in a muffin tin and fill them ¾ full. Bake at 350°F for 15 to 20 minutes.

MAKES 24 SMALL MUFFINS

Banana Bread

- 3 ripe bananas, mashed
- Juice of 1 lemon
- ½ cup honey
- ½ cup soy butter
- 1¾ cups spelt flour
- ¼ cup rice bran
- 1 teaspoon cinnamon
- ½ teaspoon baking powder
- ½ teaspoon baking soda
- ¾ cup chopped walnuts

Preheat the oven to 375°F.

Add the lemon juice to the mashed bananas in a small bowl and mix until smooth.

Mix the honey and butter together in a large bowl. Add the banana mixture and blend together.

Mix the flour, rice bran, cinnamon, baking powder, and baking soda together in a separate bowl. Fold in the walnuts. Add the dry ingredients to the liquid mixture, stirring just until blended. Pour into greased loaf pan and bake for 40 minutes at 375°F.

Let cool before cutting.

MAKES 1 LOAF

Blueberry Muffins

- 3 cups Spelt Pancake and Muffin Mix
- 1 cup skim milk
- ½ cup honey
- ½ cup fresh blueberries

Preheat the oven to 400°F.

Mix all of the ingredients together in a medium bowl until blended well. Grease the muffin tins and spoon the batter into them so they are ¾ full. Bake at 400°F for 20 minutes and let cool.

MAKES 12 MUFFINS

Spelt Bread

- 3 cups warm water
- 2 tablespoons dry, granulated yeast
- 1 tablespoon honey
- 4 cups fine spelt flour, divided
- 3 cups spelt flour

Dissolve the honey and yeast in warm water in a large bowl and stir in 1 cup fine flour. Set the bowl in a sink with very warm water until the liquid bubbles, about 15 minutes.

Using an electric mixer, beat in the remaining 3 cups of fine flour on low speed. When the flour is moist, continue beating on medium speed for 3 minutes. Gradually stir the remaining 3 cups of flour into the dough, using a large spoon. Turn the dough out on a floured board and knead for 10 minutes.

Oil a large bowl. Place the dough in it and turn once to grease the top surface of the dough. Cover with a tea towel and set in a warm place to rise.

When the dough is double in size, punch it down and knead briefly right in the bowl for 2 minutes. Cover and return to a warm place for 1 hour.

Knead on a lightly floured surface, divide, and shape into 2 loaves. Place them in oiled and floured loaf pans. Cover with a towel and put in a warm place to let the bread rise to the top of the pans.

Preheat the oven to 425°F. Remove the towel and place the bread in the oven. Bake for 15 minutes. Reduce the heat to 350°F and bake for 30 minutes more.

Remove the loaves from the pans and lay them on their sides on wire racks to cool.

MAKES 2 LOAVES

Spelt Muffins

- 2¼ cups spelt flour
- 1 tablespoon baking powder
- 1¼ cups skim milk
- 3 eggs, beaten
- ¼ cup honey
- 1 tablespoon extra-virgin olive oil
- ½ cup chopped nuts (optional)

Preheat oven to 375°F.

Combine the flour and baking powder in a large bowl. Add the milk, eggs, honey, and oil. Mix well. Add nuts if desired. Put paper muffin cups in a muffin tin and fill with batter. Bake at 375°F for 17 minutes.

MAKES 6 LARGE MUFFINS

Spelt Pie Crust

- 3 tablespoons extra-virgin olive oil
- 2 tablespoons cool water
- 1 cup plus 2 tablespoons spelt flour

Combine the oil and water in a medium bowl, and mix well. Stir in the flour and mix until evenly moistened. Press into a pie plate. Fill and bake at 350°F for 15 minutes.

Index

About the Author

Shelley Ann Smith is a pharmacy technician who suffers from fibro-myalgia. She has studied the ways in which proper eating and health habits can provide relief from the symptoms of the disease. The mother of four children, she lives in Barrie, Ontario, Canada.

Notes

Notes

Notes

Notes

Notes

Notes

Notes

_____

_____

_____

_____

_____

_____

_____

_____

_____

_____

_____

_____

_____

_____

_____

_____

_____

_____

_____

_____

_____

_____

_____

Notes

31901050588955